COPING WITH SNC

JILL ECKERSLEY is a freelance writer with many
years' experience of writing on health topics. She is a
regular contributor to womer
magazines, including *Good He*
Goodtimes, *Woman's Realm* a
beside the Regent's Canal in nor

D0283954

Overcoming Common Problems Series

A full list of titles is available from Sheldon Press,
1 Marylebone Road, London NW1 4DU, and on our website at
www.sheldonpress.co.uk

Overcoming Common Problems Series

Overcoming Common Problems Series

Overcoming Common Problems

Coping with Snoring and Sleep Apnoea

Jill Eckersley

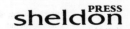

First published in Great Britain in 2003 by
Sheldon Press
1 Marylebone Road
London NW1 4DU

British Library Cataloguing-in-Publication Data
A catalogue record for this book is available from the British Library

ISBN 0–85969–890–4

1 3 5 7 9 10 8 6 4 2

Typeset by Deltatype Ltd, Birkenhead, Wirral
Printed in Great Britain by Biddles Ltd
www.biddles.co.uk

Contents

Acknowledgements

Many people have helped with the writing of this book and I should like to thank them. First, Marianne Davey of the British Snoring and Sleep Apnoea Association who answered my many questions with infinite patience – as did the many doctors I spoke to, notably Dr Peter Venn of the Sleep Studies Unit at the Queen Victoria Hospital in East Grinstead, Grant Bates of the Radcliffe Infirmary, Oxford, Michael Timms of the Abbey Gisburne Park Hospital, East Lancashire, Dr Joanna Battagel of the Royal London Hospital and Andrew Birzgalis of the Snoring Treatment Centre at BUPA's Manchester Hospital.

Thanks, too, to the many complementary practitioners who shared their expertise with me, and to Julia Cole of Relate Marriage Guidance. I should also like to thank my friends and colleagues in the Women Writers' Network who were able to put me in touch with lots of snorers and their partners and families, many of whose stories appear anonymously here. I'd like to wish all those who were brave enough to talk about their snoring problems years of uninterrupted sleep!

1

Why Snoring is No Joke

Why did you pick up this book? Perhaps you're embarrassed because someone has just told you that you snore. Perhaps you are the long-suffering partner of a snorer and you're fed up with sleepless nights, and tired of decamping to the spare room or the living-room sofa at three in the morning. Perhaps you've had enough of the jokes – because snoring really isn't funny.

Accurate figures about the number of people affected by snoring are hard to come by, but it's certain that a large minority of the UK population has a snoring problem. Globally, it has been estimated that a staggering 763 million people snore. Chinese and Afro-Caribbean people are apparently hearty snorers. In some parts of the USA, snoring is grounds for divorce, and in 1997 it was reported that an Iranian gentleman had divorced his wife for snoring.

Snoring is a problem that doesn't just affect the snorer, but his partner and family too. I say 'his' partner because more men than women snore – about 41 per cent as against 28 per cent of women, according to the British Snoring and Sleep Apnoea Association.

Dr John Rees, consultant physician and Senior Lecturer in Medicine at Guy's Hospital, says that at the moment no one really knows why men are more likely to snore than women:

> It may be related to neck size, men having larger necks in general. It may also partly relate to alcohol consumption. On top of this, the drive to respiration may generally be greater in women, especially pre-menopausal women, because of the respiratory stimulant effect of the female hormone progesterone.

By the age of 60 about half of all men are snorers, and research in Canada has recently discovered that post-menopausal women are, indeed, much more likely to snore than younger ones. This might suggest that there's a link to hormone function, with the female hormones oestrogen and progesterone having a protective effect. Another, and far simpler, reason why older women snore more is likely to be because, like older men, they tend to put on weight and lose muscle tone as they get older. The shape of women's airways is also a little different from men's. Women have slightly less flexible

1

airway walls, which don't yield to pressure in the same way. However, the British Snoring and Sleep Apnoea Association (BSSAA) do report that some older women among their members have found that being prescribed hormone replacement therapy has helped their snoring.

The fact that snoring is often much more of a problem for the listeners – partners, families and flatmates, even neighbours – than it is for the snorer can cause problems in itself. Doctors say this is one of the very few areas of medicine where they are actually treating a patient in order to benefit other people, rather than the patient himself. It is more difficult to motivate yourself to take the necessary steps to change your lifestyle, or get treatment for your snoring, if you are able to sleep sweetly through the night while your family suffer! Many snorers actually deny they have a problem, until presented with the evidence on tape. This has implications for family relationships and it's a shame to let it get to the stage where your partner is threatening to leave before you agree to do something about it. Some couples never get that far. While researching this book I came across a couple of young women who had flatly refused to move in with, or marry, the men in their lives until they had taken steps to sort out their snoring problem. I also spoke to innumerable women, and a few men, whose partners simply refused to admit that they snored, and some older people who were self-conscious about embarking on new relationships in later life because of their snoring problem.

It's embarrassing to be told you snore, just as it's embarrassing to be told you have halitosis or smelly feet. Snorers feel self-conscious and defensive about their problem, and relentless teasing from partners and flatmates is often counter-productive.

'People will mock those who snore, just as they mock anyone who falls asleep in public and laugh at politicians or public figures who make fools of themselves,' says psychologist Ken Gibbons of the Chi Health Centres, where traditional and modern medicine and psychotherapy are combined. 'Malicious humour is a very British characteristic. We like to bring people down, and although we often claim it isn't done unkindly, the effect is still hurtful.'

As far as is known, snoring doesn't run in families, although if you have inherited a short, fat neck or a particular airway anatomy from one of your parents, this may predispose you to be a snorer.

Who snores?

Everyone snores sometimes, when they have a cold or blocked nose for some other reason. A snore happens when the air you breathe hits the floppy, soft tissues at the back of the throat, which are relaxed in sleep. This leads to the rhythmic rumbling, buzzing, snuffling or grunting noises that are all too familiar to snorers and their nearest and dearest. Until very recently the loudest snores ever were recorded by researchers at Orebro University in Sweden in 1993. They measured a staggering 93 decibels (dB), as loud as a heavy lorry or passing Tube train, and were credited, if that's the right word, to a 44-year-old named Kare Walker. In the early summer of 2002, a Nottinghamshire man was said to have produced snores that hit 102 dB, roughly the same volume as an accelerating motorbike.

Ancient records reveal that some of the Roman emperors were snorers, as was Beau Brummel, the Regency dandy. In the heyday of the Wild West, it is said that legendary gunfighter John Wesley Harding became so enraged by the loud snoring of a fellow hotel guest that he shot through the wall of his room and killed him! And this isn't the only time snoring has led to murder. In 1993, Texas police arrested a woman who had shot her lover for snoring too loudly. An American truck driver, travelling to Las Vegas by bus to pick up his next rig, fell asleep on the bus and snored so loudly that the driver had to wake him up as he was disturbing the other passengers. Unfortunately he fell asleep again and had to be woken several times by the exasperated bus driver. Eventually he was hauled off the bus in handcuffs by the police and charged with disturbing the peace – the punishment being a $500 fine or six months in jail. The dangerous form of snoring, known as 'sleep apnoea', in which the subject actually stops breathing (see Chapter 7), was certainly known in the days of Charles Dickens. He describes a classic case in the overweight messenger-boy Joe in Pickwick Papers, written in 1837. Joe, described as a wonderfully fat boy who snores and breathes heavily, is advised by his master to keep knocking at the door until someone answers, in case he should fall asleep in mid-knock! Snoring, breathing heavily, and falling asleep during the daytime are all symptoms of sleep apnoea.

Distinguished snorers down the years have included Winston Churchill, who is said to have snored so loudly during the war years that his staff couldn't hear the bombs dropping on London.

Mussolini was also a snorer, as were at least 20 US presidents. When President Theodore Roosevelt was hospitalized, almost every other patient on the wing complained about his snoring. When actress Joanne Woodward was asked what it was like to be married to sex symbol Paul Newman, she replied, 'He has six children and he snores. How can he be a sex symbol?' Elizabeth Taylor is also reputed to be a snorer.

Living with a snorer

But you probably don't care about Beau Brummel . . . or Churchill . . . or even Paul Newman. All you want is a cure – and a decent night's sleep – before you're tempted to strangle the snorer in your life.

Here's Pauline, who has been married to a snorer for 18 years:

David has always snored on and off, but he has put on a bit of weight in the past year and the last six months have been a nightmare for both of us.

It's like the Chinese water torture, because even when he isn't snoring I can't relax enough to drop off because I am just waiting for him to start up. When he does it's so loud, it's like being in the middle of Grand Central Station or a farmyard. No one could be expected to sleep through it.

His snoring disturbs us both because I usually nudge him awake in the hope that changing positions will shut him up. Sometimes it does for a while . . . and then it starts again. Sometimes he kind of chokes and gasps and wakes himself up.

Like a lot of men, he hasn't yet been willing to go to our GP about it. I think he's afraid the doctor will suggest surgery. But we can't go on like this. He has tried those nasal strips that athletes wear and he did get a better night's sleep for a time. He does suffer from a stuffed-up nose and the strips seemed to keep his airway clear, but they didn't cure the noise, not really. Then I saw a dental device advertised in my local dental surgery. We splashed out over £200 on that and it didn't help much. We did have a couple of undisturbed nights but that might have been because we were both so exhausted. David said it was difficult to get used to having the device in his mouth as well.

The most serious problem it has caused is that we are both

permanently exhausted. David has a long commute to work so he really needs quality sleep. I worry about him driving when he is so tired.

I work from home, but I need my sleep as well. I've lost count of the times I've had to sleep on a fold-up bed in the study just to get away from David's snoring. It has really become an issue between us and is affecting our relationship.

And Judy, teenage daughter of another snorer:

It's embarrassing. I can't ever bring my friends home on Sundays because Dad likes to have a snooze after Sunday lunch – and believe me, you can hear him all down the street, especially in the summer when the windows are open.

When we were little we used to stay in a caravan for our holidays and it was awful, Dad kept us all awake.

Terry was quoted in a newsletter of the British Snoring and Sleep Apnoea Association (BSSAA):

When I went camping with my family, I knew I'd have to sleep in a separate tent a few feet away from my wife and children or they would never get to sleep. But I was amazed and horrified when I found a note pinned to my tent by other guests on the camping site asking me if I would mind leaving because my snoring was keeping them all awake.

Other members complain of not being able to go on holiday because the noise of snoring travels through thin holiday hotel room walls and reverberates around self-catering apartments or campsites. Many are too embarrassed to go away to stay with friends or invite them to stay for a weekend.

'Holidays are a huge problem for snorers and their families,' comments Marianne Davey of the BSSAA:

At least when they are at home, partners can escape to the sofa or, if they're lucky, the spare room. Few people have the resources to be able to afford separate rooms on holiday. We always advise snorers to contact us three months before they plan to go away so that we can offer them some solutions in plenty of time!

Liz has been a victim of snoring for most of her life. 'I've heard all the jokes but believe me, it isn't funny,' she says:

> My parents were both really bad snorers and slept separately for years. It made them very irritable with each other and divorce was threatened at least three times, though they did stay together in the end.
>
> I never thought that I would marry a snorer, but my husband has put on a lot of weight in the years we've been together and I now have to wear earplugs because of his snoring. Luckily I only work part-time. If I had a demanding full-time job and children to look after, it would kill me.
>
> My husband is a typical man in that he would really rather ignore health problems and becomes defensive if I mention his snoring. I have to pick my moment or he just refuses to discuss it. He has tried most of the over-the-counter so-called 'cures' but they were useless. When I finally persuaded him to go to the doctor, he was told there was nothing that could be done for him. I'm sure that can't be right.
>
> We used to live in a one-bed flat and I spent most of my time sleeping on the sofa. It did nothing for our love life – in fact we didn't have one. But we have recently moved to a three-bedroom house which we deliberately chose so that we could have separate rooms if we wanted. I'm also hoping that our new GP will be more up-to-date about what can be done. I've heard there's an operation you can have.
>
> At the moment I am trying to help my husband to lose weight and take more exercise, maybe join a gym, but I have to pick my moment to suggest anything like that.

Alan's marriage actually broke up as a direct result of his snoring problem. 'My wife couldn't stand it any more,' he admits:

> I was turning into a slob, a complete couch potato. I was always so tired that as soon as I sat down after dinner I fell asleep. It was like being permanently jet-lagged. I had no energy or desire to do anything, even things I used to enjoy, like gardening. I did try to lose weight and managed to shed a couple of stone, but it wasn't easy as I was going out for business lunches and then coming home to a nice meal in the evening. When you feel as lethargic as I did, exercise is the last thing you feel like doing.

6

After my marriage broke up my GP sent me for a 'sleep study' and I was diagnosed with sleep apnoea, the most serious form of snoring. I was told that while I was asleep I actually stopped breathing about 80 times a hour, and if I didn't do something about it I had about a 50-per-cent chance of dying of asphyxiation. Sadly, it was too late to save my marriage, but at least my life is no longer at risk.

Snoring and health

Snoring isn't an illness, but it is a symptom – of anything from the common cold to a more serious respiratory problem. Snorers seem generally to be less healthy than non-snorers. Research suggests that snorers have a higher than average risk of developing high blood pressure, heart attacks or stroke illness. A recent study conducted at the University of Buffalo, New York, found that people who experience disturbed sleep patterns are twice as likely to suffer strokes as those who sleep straight through the night. A study of about 500 70-year-olds in Denmark in the 1980s found that:

- blood pressure was about 15 per cent higher in snorers than it was in people who didn't snore;
- 11 per cent of the snorers suffered from angina, compared with only 5 per cent of the non-snorers;
- 15 per cent of the snorers had symptoms of arterial disease in their legs, compared with only 6 per cent of the non-snorers.

These results were adjusted for factors like body weight and smoking. According to Dr Rees of Guy's Hospital, researchers over the last few years have been trying to discover whether snorers are at risk of high blood pressure, heart attacks and strokes because they are snorers, or because they also tend to be overweight smokers and drinkers, all risk factors for these conditions. About 10 per cent of snorers go on to develop a potentially fatal condition called 'obstructive sleep apnoea' – for more about this, see Chapter 7.

'There is now good evidence that obstructive sleep apnoea and possibly even snoring itself are related to high blood pressure, heart attacks and strokes independently of the association with weight, smoking and drinking,' he says. 'The risk of these problems for snorers is not huge, but seems definitely to exist.'

The most obvious health problems caused by snoring are those associated with fatigue, which include anxiety, irritability, and poor memory and concentration. These, in their turn, can lead to problems at work and at home. No one is at their most efficient when they are chronically exhausted, and that means lower productivity as well as real danger for anyone whose job depends on alertness, from doctors to drivers. It's estimated that about 10 per cent of car crashes are caused by tired drivers. Daytime sleepiness obviously affects a person's ability to do their job properly, and in the evening they are usually too tired to take a normal part in family and social life, preferring to nod off in front of the TV.

Lack of sleep also affects emotional health. Tired people are not happy people, and sleeplessness can turn a normally loving partner or concerned parent into a bad-tempered grouch with no time or sympathy for friends or family.

There is no one-size-fits-all, guaranteed cure for snoring, no 'magic bullet' that will suddenly turn a snorer into a silent sleeping partner! But there are treatments, and there are ways of managing the condition. Some just involve simple lifestyle changes, others are more complex. There is no need to despair, however long you have suffered, because help is available, both for snorers and for their partners.

The Surrey-based British Snoring and Sleep Apnoea Association was set up in 1991 as a self-help group for snorers and their families. Founder and director Marianne Davey says:

> Thirty years ago there seemed to be no research at all in this country, though America was about ten years ahead. If you went to your GP with the problem you would probably just be told you had to put up with it. Recently there has been an explosion of interest from doctors, dentists and maxillofacial consultants. GPs still get no training in the subject, although some have a particular interest. Many will refer you to your local ear, nose and throat (ENT) department. In good health authorities though, ENT, chest clinics and maxillofacial departments all work together. Once you know the cause of your snoring you can be referred for the most appropriate treatment.

Is there a typical snorer?

Can you spot a snorer? He is most likely to be male, middle-aged or older, and overweight, but, confusingly, he may be none of those things. Younger people and even some children snore too.

'I always thought of snorers as sad, fat gits,' says Melanie, whose thirtysomething boyfriend was acutely embarrassed when she told him he snored:

> But Peter isn't like that at all – he's fit, good-looking, goes to the gym, but still he snores. We have a good relationship and have been together for eight years but snoring is a bit of a taboo subject for us. It affects things like going on holiday. I need my sleep, but it's really difficult to raise the topic of having separate rooms in our holiday hotel – not to mention the expense.

In January 2002 American researchers reported that people whose heads were round rather than narrow were at greater risk of snoring. They had looked at 60 snorers and 60 non-snorers and compared head shapes using X-rays.

'As the head gets relatively wider, the airway becomes relatively narrower, front to back,' says Dr Mark Hans, Chair of Orthodontics at Case Western Reserve School of Dentistry.

The shape of your head or jaw, the thickness of your neck, the size of your tonsils, adenoids and uvula (the flap of skin at the back of your throat) can all influence whether you snore or not. These aren't things you would necessarily be aware of, or be able to do anything about, any more than you can help your age or your sex. You might be aware of a nasal obstruction, although without sophisticated medical tests it would be hard to work out exactly where it was. You might also know you had a particularly short lower jaw. However, there are plenty of other factors you *can* do something about, like being overweight, smoking and drinking. Snoring is just as much a lifestyle as it is a medical issue. Even if you decide to enlist the help of your doctor and experts like the BSSAA, you'll almost certainly have to make some lifestyle changes if you are serious about becoming a non-snorer. That's the not-so-good news. The good news is that you and your family don't have to suffer. What you have to do, first of all, is establish exactly why you snore . . .

2

What Happens When You Snore

Human beings were not designed to snore. We are pretty much the only mammals who do, probably because few animals sleep on their backs. It was probably when our simian ancestors started sleeping on their backs that snoring problems began. Sleeping curled up on your stomach or on your side allows your jaw to fall forward so that you're more likely to breathe normally.

Healthy non-snorers breathe through their noses. The air passes almost silently, straight over the soft palate and down the throat into the lungs. When any part of this upper airway – mouth, nose or throat – is blocked or partially blocked, snoring can result. The sound of snoring is actually the sound of the soft tissues of the airway vibrating as air passes over them. In the daytime, when we are awake, our muscles work to hold the airways open. That's why we don't snore when we're awake. During sleep, though, all our muscles relax, including the muscles of the mouth, nose and throat. The airway narrows and sags inwards as we breathe in. This combination of narrowed airways and a blockage caused by swollen soft tissue, congestion caused by a cold or allergic reactions, or sometimes by the shape of the jaw or nasal passages themselves, results in the sound of snoring.

If you think of your throat as a collapsible tube, the muscles at the base of your tongue are holding it open while you are awake. When you sleep, these muscles relax and your throat collapses. Most people still retain enough muscle tone to keep their airways clear enough to breathe properly, but if there is a lot of fatty tissue in your throat, the air flow will be impeded. As the 'tube' becomes smaller, the air currents passing through become more turbulent, resulting in snoring.

Working out why you snore

Before you can find an effective treatment for your snoring, it's essential to work out *why* you snore. Sometimes the reason will be obvious. You have a heavy cold and your head feels as if it is stuffed with catarrh. Once you've recovered, your nose will clear, you will no longer breathe through your mouth and your breathing will return to normal. However, your reason for snoring could be something more complex and it could also be the result of a combination of factors that all need investigation.

Age, weight and sex

Age, weight and sex are all significant. The older you are, the more likely you are to snore. This is because the muscles of your throat, like your other muscles, become less efficient with age. Middle-aged spread doesn't just affect your middle: flabby muscles in your throat can be a problem too. It has even been suggested that professional singers are unlikely to snore, because of the workout their throat muscles get, though sadly there seems to be no real scientific evidence for this.

Being overweight is a major contributory factor. Most experts claim that, for men, a collar size of 17 or over practically guarantees snoring. Excess fat, round your neck and throat especially, is sure to narrow those air passages and lead to snoring. In the USA it's estimated that about half the adult population is obese, and the UK seems to be going the same way. With more and more of us becoming seriously overweight – it's predicted that by 2010 more than 50 per cent of Britons will be more than 25-per-cent over weight – it rather looks as though we are in for an epidemic of noisy nights.

Smoking, alcohol and drugs

Smokers are more likely to snore than non-smokers, and passive smoking – breathing in other people's smoke – can also have an effect, especially on children. Cigarette, pipe and cigar smoke irritates the lining of the nose and can lead to a build-up of catarrh and congestion in the nasal passages. Once your nose is congested you are more likely to breathe through your mouth, and the result is more snoring.

Alcohol and sleeping pills can also have an effect on snoring. Alcohol is a depressant that causes the muscles to relax, including the throat muscles, leading to even more narrowed airways and more snoring. Studies in Australia have shown that even moderate alcohol consumption can affect the way we breathe and the amount we snore. Even after what most of us would describe as 'social drinking', people who normally snored harmlessly suffered from periods of the more dangerous sleep apnoea in the first two hours of sleep.

In other words, you don't have to be drunk to have breathing problems. The Australian researchers measured the amount of oxygen in the blood of snorers who had been drinking. The blood of healthy individuals normally has 100 per cent oxygen saturation. In snorers the levels were 89 per cent on average, and in snorers who had been drinking, oxygen levels dropped to 73 per cent or even lower. Without a constant and regular supply of oxygen in your blood, all your tissues will suffer, most significantly your heart and your brain, leading, in the worst cases, to heart attacks and strokes. Since the majority of snorers are overweight middle-aged men who are already at increased risk of these problems, snoring compounds their risk.

Some sleeping pills have a similar effect. According to Dr John Rees of Guy's Hospital, most of the hypnotics or sleeping pills that are prescribed can make both snoring and sleep apnoea worse because they depress breathing to some degree. Most of the studies have been done on commonly used drugs like the benzodiazepines, of which Valium is an example. As well as being prescribed to treat anxiety and anxiety-related insomnia, Valium is known to be a muscle relaxant and, as we have learned, relaxed throat muscles mean more snoring.

People who are already snorers and who drink heavily are more likely to develop sleep apnoea, the dangerous form of snoring where breathing stops altogether, leading to more health complications.

Sleeping position

The position you sleep in can also play a part. People who sleep on their backs are more likely to snore as their tongues fall back into their throats, causing an obstruction. Again, the overweight are at more risk because excess fat under the chin can also narrow the airway if you sleep on your back.

Allergies

Allergic-type conditions such as hay fever and a reaction to house-dust mites in your bedding can also cause a congested nose and that 'stuffy' feeling, similar to a head cold. Even your diet can be implicated. Some people find that over-consumption of dairy products leads to excessive mucus in the nose and throat. All the air you breathe has to pass through the nasal valve area at the back of each nostril. This nasal valve is only 2·54 mm ($\frac{1}{10}$ inch) wide so is very easily blocked.

Physical features

Physical features can play a part too. The shape of your jaw and the width of your nostrils, nasal growths or polyps, a particularly large soft palate, tongue or uvula (the flap of skin you can see at the back of your throat when you open your mouth wide) or a deviated septum (an abnormality in the cartilage that divides the nostrils) might be the cause of your problem. Any or all of these can cause obstructed breathing, especially if you breathe through your mouth. Apparently, experts in sleep study clinics can often tell from the sound of snoring whether the problem originates in your palate or your nose, or whether it's caused by your tongue falling back as you sleep and blocking the airway. This is a good argument for tape-recording your snoring if you find that simple lifestyle changes, like losing weight or changing your sleeping position, seem to have no effect.

Less common causes

There are other, less common reasons for snoring. One of them, curiously, is pregnancy. Hormone changes during this time soften all your muscles in preparation for the birth, and softer throat muscles mean more snoring. At least if that is your problem, you know it's likely to right itself after the birth!

As a complete contrast, the anabolic steroids taken by some body-builders to build up muscle tissue have much the same effect, according to some experts, with nandrolone being a particular offender. Would-be musclemen should take note. Sleepless nights, irritability and damaged relationships could be too high a price to pay for bulging biceps.

People with high blood pressure are also more likely to be snorers.

Getting to the root of the problem

It's quite likely that several of these factors could apply to you at the same time. Snoring doesn't always have a simple cause. To get to the root of the problem you will need to ask yourself questions like:

- When did you start to snore, or when did you or your partner feel that snoring had become a problem?
- Had you made any lifestyle changes? For instance, was your

alcohol intake creeping up, had you started on a course of sleeping tablets or other prescription drugs, had you changed your diet or put on weight in the last few months?

- Do you use street drugs? Opiates like heroin and cocaine are also likely to make snoring worse.
- Do you have any other allergic symptoms, such as hay fever?

What is making you snore?

Snoring isn't a disease, it's a lifestyle issue, and lifestyle factors are usually implicated even when there turns out to be a physical reason for your snoring, like the shape of your jaw or the size of your uvula or tongue, as well.

The tongue is a muscle, and like any muscle it can become loose and floppy. You might also have a larger-than-average tongue, or a narrower-than-average airway, or both. The BSSAA recommends a series of tests that you can apply to discover whether your problem is your tongue, your palate, the shape of your nostrils, or whether you are a 'mouth breather', so that you (and your doctor) can select the most appropriate treatment.

Many of the over-the-counter snoring remedies you can buy are aimed at clearing stuffed-up nostrils. If this is the reason for your snoring, you will be aware of it, and a nasal spray may help. It's very important that you look for the cause of the stuffiness and treat that, rather than relying on treating the symptoms.

To find out whether or not it's your tongue that is causing the problem, try this test, devised by the BSSAA. If you are able to make a snoring sound with your mouth both open and closed, stick your tongue out as far as you possibly can and grip it between your teeth. Now try and repeat the snoring sound. If the sound is reduced when you are holding your tongue in this 'forward' position, then you are probably a tongue-based snorer.

Another specially devised BSSAA test is designed to identify mouth breathers who sleep with their mouths open, causing snoring. Normally, breathing through the nose ensures that the air passes gently over the palate and into the throat. if you breathe through your mouth, the air hits the back of the throat head on, causing the soft tissues to vibrate. Try this test. Open your mouth and make a snoring noise. Now close your mouth and try again. If you only snore when your mouth is open you're a mouth breather, and any treatment should involve helping you to keep your mouth closed when you sleep and to breathe correctly, through your nose.

Snoring and children

Snoring in children and young people is not common, but not unknown. It often goes unnoticed for some time because parents, unlike partners, are not often kept awake at night by snoring youngsters. However, children who seem to suffer from more colds than average or permanently stuffed-up noses may also snore at night. A spokesman for the Royal College of Paediatrics and Child Health says that it's a good idea for the parents of children who seem to have breathing difficulties to spend 10 or 15 minutes outside the child's bedroom to listen to their breathing. If there seem to be a lot of pauses, grunts and snuffles – and snoring – it is worth checking it out with your GP.

'Snoring is a rare phenomenon in children but it does exist,' he says:

By far the most common reason for breathing difficulties in children is an allergy, often to house-dust mites, pet hair or cigarette smoke. A few children might have some congenital abnormality of the airway but that would be obvious to both parents and doctors. Another possible cause is enlarged adenoids. A very tiny proportion of the children who snore are actually suffering from sleep apnoea – the condition in which they stop breathing altogether for a few seconds – perhaps because they have very large tonsils and adenoids.

Parents whose children snore should consult their GP, as it is unusual. In nine out of ten cases the child will have a swollen nasal lining due to an allergy, and may also be asthmatic or suffer from eczema. Initial treatment would probably be similar to that offered to an adult with nasal congestion – either anti-histamines, nasal steroids or sodium cromoglicate 'Rynacrom', a standard hay fever type of drug. If this doesn't work then enlarged adenoids might be suspected and the child would be referred to an ENT surgeon to consider the possibility of surgery to remove them. This operation isn't done anything like as frequently as it used to be, and most surgeons are reluctant to operate unless it's absolutely necessary.

If the child is found to be suffering from sleep apnoea – they are very sleepy during the day, keep choking and gasping for breath and waking up in the night – then the tonsils and adenoids will probably have to be removed. Only a very small number of children would need this kind of surgery.

According to recent research in the USA and Finland, untreated sleep apnoea can sometimes result in a slower-than-normal growth rate, plus behaviour and heart problems in children. This is probably because such children never get a chance to sleep really deeply and it's in the 'deep' stages of sleep that growth hormone is released. One survey from Kentucky looked at 1,500 children and found that only 5 per cent of the high achievers had snored in early childhood, compared with 13 per cent of those who did less well at school. The Director of the Paediatric Sleep Medicine Centre at Arkansas Children's Hospital says that sleep-deprived children tend to exhibit oppositional behaviour, and have short attention spans and an inability to focus on school work that sometimes results in their being misdiagnosed with Attention Deficit Hyperactivity Disorder. British paediatricians don't, at present, believe that snoring actually causes behavioural difficulties, even though a small proportion of 'disturbed' children do suffer from sleep apnoea. In any case, snoring in children definitely requires investigation.

The BSSAA also hear from parents concerned about snoring children and say that they have found allergies to be the chief cause, along with passive smoking. Apparently it's not enough, if you're a smoking parent, simply to avoid smoking in your child's bedroom or when you're with the child. Even a small amount of tobacco smoke in the house can have a measurable effect on an allergic child. The Royal College of Paediatrics recommends that if you have a family history of allergic illness, ranging from asthma and eczema to hay fever, it's best to make sure you have a smoke- and pet-free home before you even plan a pregnancy.

Thinking carefully about your lifestyle, and applying the BSSAA tests on p. 14 should give you a good idea of what is making you snore. It probably won't be just one thing – you may be overweight *and* sleep on your back *and* be allergic to house-dust mites or cigarette smoke. Before you even approach your GP for help, it's a good idea to consider some basic lifestyle changes. The BSSAA say that if you can manage to reduce your $17\frac{1}{2}$ collar size to $16\frac{1}{2}$ you (and your nearest and dearest) could notice quite a difference in your snoring pattern. Why not give it a try?

3

Simple Cures and Lifestyle Changes

Before you can make a serious attempt to tackle your snoring, you really do need to work out why you snore. What you have read already should have given you some clues, and after that it is largely a matter of working through all the possibilities before you can decide on an effective remedy or remedies.

Simple solutions

Sleeping position

Most snorers' partners begin by giving them a dig in the ribs and this can be effective, if uncomfortable, on a temporary basis at least. It will usually make the snorer shift position. Remember, it's often sleeping on your back, with your mouth open, that leads to problems, so anything that can help you into another sleeping position may do the trick. You could try stitching a tennis ball or even a clothes peg into the back of your pyjamas – but success is not guaranteed.

A more comfortable version of the same idea is to sleep with pillows in the small of your back, which will make it more difficult for you to flop over in the night. Some people swear by raising the head of the bed slightly. If you are lying on your back it is much more likely that your tongue, relaxed in sleep, will fall to the back of your throat. This is what causes snoring in tongue-based snorers. If you can manage to sleep through your snoring and your partner can't, let your partner go to bed an hour earlier so that they are well away before you begin to snore.

Nasal congestion

If you decide that nasal congestion is the root of your problem, do you know what is causing it? A simple cold will clear up within a week, so if the catarrh lasts for longer than that you could have a more complex problem. Could an allergy be to blame? Are you suffering from hay fever? Some people find that inhaling steam is a good way to recondition their nasal passages. Just pour some boiling water into a basin – you can add a small amount of a decongestant like Vick if you like – and lean over with a towel over your head for ten minutes, morning and evening, breathing in the steam. If this has no effect, ask your pharmacist or GP about anti-histamines or other treatments like cortico-steroids.

House-dust mites, which live in their thousands in even the cleanest bedding and carpets, release allergens that cause nasal stuffiness and catarrh in susceptible people. Up to 5,000 dust mites can live in a single gram of house dust and they thrive in warm, poorly ventilated houses. Allergy UK, formerly known as the British Allergy Foundation (see p. 83), can offer tips and hints on how to combat the problem. Among their recommendations are:

- Increase the ventilation in your home by leaving windows open whenever possible.
- Turn down the central heating, especially in bedrooms.
- Reduce humidity – don't dry washing indoors, and keep the bathroom door closed when running a bath. Reduce steam by running the cold water in first.
- Use an extractor fan or ventilated cooker hood when cooking, or keep the kitchen window open.
- Use allergy-free bed-linen and mattress covers, which you can buy from some chemists and specialist retailers as well as department stores. Companies like Medivac and Medibed (see pp. 83–84) produce air-permeable covers for mattresses, duvets and pillows. They are made of a special closely woven fabric that allergens cannot penetrate, but are still cool and comfortable to the skin, and many allergy sufferers find them of great benefit.
- Wash all bed-linen at 60 degrees.
- Use a damp cloth for dusting.
- Turn your mattress and vacuum it monthly. Avoid padded headboards.
- Consider replacing carpets with wood or vinyl floors and heavy curtains with blinds.
- Keep pets off furniture and out of bedrooms.
- Use a vacuum cleaner with a HEPA (high-energy particulate air) filter – Allergy UK have a list of approved models, which include some of the Henry, Dyson, Miele and Panasonic ranges. These vacuum cleaners are specially designed to filter the air coming out of the exhaust so that there is no release of allergens, and most dust mites and pollen are filtered out. Water-filtered models are

available as well – check with Allergy UK and major electrical retailers for the latest models. The Medivap Automatic, for example (available from Medivac) uses ordinary tap water to generate steam which can be used on upholstery, carpets, mattresses and clothes, and has been proven in medical trials to eliminate the allergens caused by dust mites.

Taking some or all of these simple steps might be enough by themselves to cure your snoring, or at least reduce it to a manageable level.

Tape-recording your snoring

The BSSAA also recommends tape-recording your snoring. There are considerable benefits to doing this – especially if you are the kind of snorer who still isn't convinced you have a problem! Your partner will probably be only too relieved to co-operate. You can buy voice-activated tape recorders, similar in style to the Walkman, that you can set to begin recording as soon as the noise reaches a certain level. If you are referred to a sleep clinic or a consultant, you will then be able to present them with the evidence. Expert researchers can apparently tell from the frequency levels of snoring noise whether the sounds are made by the snorer's tongue or soft palate, which obviously has implications for the effectiveness of any treatment prescribed.

Lifestyle changes

The simplest lifestyle changes you can make that will have an effect on your snoring are to lose weight, give up smoking and moderate your alcohol intake. If you are referred to an ENT department or sleep studies unit by your GP, these will be the first pieces of advice you are given before any other treatments are even considered. Because these are simple steps, that's not to say they're easy, as anyone who has tried to get fit and stay healthy for other reasons knows.

The Boots company runs 'lifestyle programmes' that include Quit Smoking, Managing Your Weight and Getting Beyond Stress at selected stores in London, Birmingham, Manchester, Leeds, Oxford, Cambridge, Reading, Milton Keynes and Tunbridge Wells. Call 0845 120 3000 for more details.

Losing weight

Obesity is one of the most common reasons for snoring. Inside every overweight smoker there's a lean, fit, healthy non-smoker and non-snorer, struggling to get out! What you have to do is alter your mindset to allow the person you could be the chance to escape.

It's easy to get hold of one of those 'ideal weight' tables that tell you how heavy you should be. There's no point in cheating yourself. If you can pinch 2.5 cm (1 inch) or more of flab around your stomach, thighs or upper arms, you could probably do with losing a few kilos. To be strictly accurate about it, calculate your BMI, or 'body mass index' (you will need to be a mathematician, or use a calculator). To work out your BMI, divide your weight in kilos by your height in metres, squared. A man weighing 70k (11st) who is 1.76m tall (5ft 9in) has a BMI of 22.6 (70 divided by 1.76 x 1.76). This a perfectly healthy measurement. The BMI of a healthy man should be between 20 and 25 and a healthy woman between 19 and 24. If your BMI is over 30, you are officially obese, and having a BMI between 25 and 30 means you should lose some weight.

Think positive

Don't think in terms of 'going on a diet'. If you do you will begin to feel resentful and deprived before you have even started and, hey presto, you'll be pigging out on chocolate bars, Big Macs or whatever your particular weakness is before you know it. Losing weight is as much a matter of the right psychology as the right eating plan.

Think positive instead. You are going to get fit and healthy. Not only will this help with your snoring problem, but there will be dozens of other health benefits too. You'll feel better. You'll sleep better. You'll be able to run for a bus, take part in sports or a bit of rough-and-tumble with the kids in the park. You'll have masses more energy because you won't be carrying around all that extra lard. It's estimated that a 10-per-cent weight loss can have a significant effect on snoring patterns. If becoming a non-snorer isn't sufficient incentive for you to lose that excess weight, remind yourself of the health risks of obesity.

- Someone who is 20 per cent overweight runs a 25-per-cent higher risk of premature death.
- Someone who is 30 per cent overweight runs a 50-per-cent higher risk of early death.

- A man who is even 10 per cent overweight runs a 13-per-cent higher risk of early death.
- Obese women are at slightly less risk of early death than obese men – sorry, guys!

How to lose weight

How to do it? Well, there are literally dozens of 'diet' books and plans available. If you are seriously overweight – say, more than 20 per cent heavier than you should be for your height – a visit to your GP is in order.

In spite of what the multi-million pound slimming industry would have us believe, there's really only one way to lose weight and keep it off, and that is to:

1 eat less; and
2 exercise more.

Simple, isn't it? Most of us make excuses, saying that it's in our genes or we have a slow metabolism. Even more of us are fooled into trying peculiar fad diets involving matching your food intake to your blood group, eating loads of grapefruit or replacing normal, healthy meals with yucky-tasting milk shakes or dried cabbage soup. Diets like that don't work in the long term, mainly because they are so boring and/or unpleasant that people just can't wait to get to the end of the regime and then head off to the chippie or the Indian takeaway.

No, the only way to lose weight healthily and permanently is to re-educate your palate to enjoy sensible portions of good, healthy food. Go easy on fats and sugars, which just provide empty calories, and fill up on wholemeal bread and pasta, not forgetting your five portions of fruit and veg a day.

Don't even try to starve yourself. If you fancy a biscuit, don't beat yourself up about it, just have one – only don't polish off the entire packet, and remind yourself to snack on an apple or a handful of grapes next time. It has never been easier to eat healthily. You can save calories by grilling rather than frying, replacing full-fat milk with skimmed or semi-skimmed, replacing butter with low-fat spreads and puddings with fresh fruit. Do it gradually and you will hardly notice!

Change your thinking

Sports psychologist and personal trainer Pete Cohen, founder of the Lighten Up workshops that have helped hundreds of people to lose weight successfully and have a healthy relationship with food, believes that changing the way you think about diet and exercise is the key to success. Here are some of his tips.

- Use the Hunger Scale. When you're tempted to snack, ask yourself how hungry you really are – on a scale of 1 to 10. If the answer is less than 5, do something else instead.
- Think before you eat. How will you feel about what you've just eaten in a hour's time?
- Eat slowly so that you really savour your food. Put down your knife and fork in between mouthfuls. It takes a little time for your brain to signal to your stomach that you have had enough. Give it a chance to work!
- Eat only when you are hungry and stop when you have had enough.
- Wait five minutes, or more, in between courses. If you are already full, you don't need a pudding, cheese, a liqueur or an after-dinner mint.

The Lighten Up organization now runs special sessions for men, because they found that men approach the whole business of dieting in a different way from women.

'Men are less obsessed with the shape of their bodies,' says spokeswoman Judith Verity:

They don't worry about food all the time, unlike women, many of whom can't eat normally at all because they are so obsessional.

We found that when men get to a certain age, which may be as young as 30, they just give up on their bodies altogether. They might see that their friends are putting on weight but somehow they don't relate it to themselves. In a sense, a man will 'delete' his body and go on buying the same size trousers, even though he now has to button them up beneath his increasing tummy!

Men are sold the heavy-drinking, high-living lifestyle and somehow they don't associate the four pints of beer and the large helping of chips with their weight increase. And men, unlike women, tend to prefer exercise if it's competitive. They enjoy team games, or they will jog if they're training for a team or a special event.

They need to be motivated to lose weight. One way is what I

call the 'Scrooge' exercise, where I ask them to imagine what they will look like in a year's time if they don't lose that weight. Other men come along because they are already motivated – one man has caught a glimpse of his beer belly in a mirror, another has made a fool of himself in the dads' race at his son's school sports, another is divorced and daren't spend a night with a new girlfriend because of his snoring. Once you get the mindset right, the rest follows.

Exercise

Eating less is only half the story. You will also need to increase the amount of exercise you do. As well as helping you to lose weight, a sensible exercise regime will help you to sleep more soundly. Why not get your partner to join you in your new exercise regime? If your snoring has led to sleepless nights for both of you, exercise can help to put things right. Exercise is also known to lift depression by increasing the production of endorphins, the body's feel-good hormones – so what are you waiting for?

The vital thing is to choose a kind of exercise you like, or you will be tempted to give up. It may be fashionable to join a gym or lift weights, but if you hate it you won't keep going and it won't do your body (or your pocket) any good at all.

You can start by incorporating more exercise into your everyday routine. Walk or cycle to work or to the shops. Use the stairs at work instead of the lift. Go for a walk after Sunday lunch instead of settling down for a snooze in your favourite armchair. Aim for a minimum of half an hour's exercise a day, every day, and more if you can manage it. Household chores, from scrubbing the kitchen floor or mowing the lawn to cleaning the car and gardening, can be good exercise too. Or you could try swimming, yoga, T'ai Chi, bowls, jogging, dancing, squash, badminton, keep fit, archery, golf, skipping, trampolining, Pilates or working out to a fitness video – the list is endless. You should be aware, however, that 'spot-reduction' is not really possible. In other words, your new fitness regime will help you to a trimmer, more toned body, and losing some excess fat round your neck will be part of that. Sadly, there is no known exercise regime that will enable you to lose weight from the neck area alone.

Giving up smoking

Like losing weight, giving up smoking will pay dividends health-wise as well as helping your snoring problem. (You'll feel the difference in your wallet or purse too!) Since the link between smoking and lung cancer was made public in the early 1960s, more and more people have managed to give up and fewer than a third of British adults now smoke. You could, as well. You have probably heard hundreds of times that smokers are at higher risk of cancer, heart attacks, strokes and other respiratory diseases, and that women who smoke risk miscarriage, low birthweight babies, cervical cancer, etc., etc., etc. Most smokers want to give up, but nicotine is a highly addictive substance, and for many it isn't easy and can take several attempts. Nicotine patches or gum, worry beads to fiddle with or hypnosis all work for some people. Others just go 'cold turkey', stub out their final cigarette and put the money they have saved towards their next holiday. Contact Quitline (see p. 84) for more details of how you, too, could become a non-smoker.

Cutting down on alcohol

If you suspect that alcohol could be a factor in your snoring, try reducing your intake and see what happens. You don't have to be a very heavy drinker to feel the effects. Australian research has shown that alcohol:

- relaxes the muscles of the airway;
- depresses the 'respiratory drive' in the brain that keeps us breathing regularly even when we sleep;
- slows up the 'waking response', which normally wakes us up when something interferes with our regular breathing.

Some experts recommend that anyone who snores very heavily or has been diagnosed as suffering from sleep apnoea should abstain from alcohol in the evenings altogether. In any case, if your snoring is drink-related it makes sense to cut down on alcohol, perhaps alternating alcoholic and non-alcoholic drinks in social situations. If alcohol is a factor in your snoring, the BSSAA recommends leaving a four-hour gap between drinking alcohol and going to bed.

Simple steps: Brian and Laura

Brian and Laura found that simple steps were sufficient to nip their snoring problems in the bud, before the subject became an issue between them. Laura says:

> I wouldn't say either of us snored really badly, or not compared to some of the couples we knew, who were always sniping at one another about it. But we did both snore, and I noticed that with Brian it was usually after he had been out for a few pints with his friends. He was beginning to develop a beer belly, too. As for me, I'd put on weight after I had the children and never seemed to be able to lose it. At first I sort of accepted it as part of getting older but then I thought no, we're only in our forties, maybe we should do something about it.
>
> We planned to take up jogging, and we gave it a go, but we found it boring. A friend of mine was going to a yoga class and although I wasn't sure about it at first, I found it really, really relaxing. I don't know whether all the breathing exercises helped me not to snore, or whether it was making changes to the family diet so we ate fewer cakes and puddings and more fruit and vegetables, but the effect was that I lost a stone without really trying.
>
> It turned out Brian had been a bit worried about the amount he was drinking anyway, so he was glad to have an excuse to cut down. He walks part of the way to work and restricts his drinking to two or three nights a week. He drinks halves now, not pints. He looks and feels better and hardly ever snores – or if he does I don't hear him!

If you're lucky, lifestyle changes may be enough by themselves to solve your snoring problem, and they will bring additional benefits too. You'll both look and feel better and that will improve your self-esteem. If your snoring has been affecting your relationship, at least your partner will see that you are trying to do something about it. However, if you're not a 'typical snorer' – you're a normal weight for your height, and you don't smoke or drink – you must begin to suspect that your nose and throat are becoming congested for other reasons. Perhaps some of the 'clinically proven' wonder-cures you see on the shelves of your local chemist's shop would be worth a try. Do they really work? There's often only one way to find out . . .

4

Snoring Remedies – Will They Work for You?

You've tried the dig-in-the-ribs method. You're eating sensibly and maybe you have already lost some weight. You've stopped smoking and are going easy on the alcohol – but you're still snoring. If you go into your local chemist you will see a variety of products and devices all claiming to 'cure snoring', from odd-looking plastic things you put up your nose to pills, mouthwashes and throat sprays with apparently magic ingredients that claim to be 'clinically proven' to do the trick and lead to silent, snore-free nights.

Do any of them work? The best that can be said is that some products give some people some help, some of the time.

Choosing the right remedy

You always have to remember that the causes of snoring are many and varied. If you buy a product that is not tailored for your individual problem the results are likely to disappoint you. Sprays designed to cure nasal congestion will not help if your snoring is caused by the shape of your jaw, or the way your tongue falls to the back of your throat when you sleep. Few over-the-counter products give much information about the kind of snoring they are designed to cure. Your pharmacist may be able to help you with advice, though many rely on the information supplied by the manufacturer. My own, totally unscientific, survey found that local independent pharmacies carried a wider range of anti-snoring remedies than the major chains like Boots and Superdrug. A wide variety of earplugs is also available in the High Street, some simple foam devices, others made of a wax-like substance that moulds to your ears.

In December 2001, *Health Which?*, the consumer magazine, put a variety of anti-snoring products to the test. They gave eight couples anti-snoring products to try, and recorded the results, both for the snorers and for their partners. They also took a look at the products from a medical point of view. Most claimed to be 'clinically proven' to cure or at least reduce snoring, but a more detailed look at the research behind the claims showed that some of it was flawed. In some cases, the numbers of snorers in the trial were so small that the results weren't statistically significant. Of course, exactly the same criticism could be levelled at the *Health Which?* tests, since only one couple was asked to test each product. In other cases the clinical trials weren't 'blind' and snorers actually knew which product they were trying.

This doesn't, of course, mean that these products don't work for individuals, just that you should always take manufacturers' claims with a pinch of salt. The BSSAA say that you should be extremely wary of any product which claims that it is 'guaranteed' to cure snoring, without being more specific about who it is designed to help. If you are still grossly overweight, still smoking, still drinking heavily, then many over-the-counter snoring remedies won't help at all. For instance, very few 'cures' will actually tell you whether they are suitable for nose-based, tongue-based or palate-based snorers. One of the *Which?* experts, a senior lecturer in restorative dentistry, felt that all anti-snoring products should carry a warning that snoring should be investigated by a physician before any products are tried.

'All the products we sell are clinically proven to help some snorers,' says Marianne Davey of the BSSAA:

> Before we take a product on board or recommend it to members, we ask to see the research and the evidence and we do our own tests as well. Sometimes we hear of people buying 'cures' from shops or over the Web, and of course they get no back-up. The sellers are not snoring experts and are not really equipped to advise people about the products they sell. Although we do sell anti-snoring remedies we never pressurize anyone to buy. Our strength lies in giving advice and information to snorers about what may help in their individual case. For example, some snorers who have a problem with nasal congestion find that nasal dilators fall out, and we may be able to recommend Breathe Right strips which could suit them better. Or snorers who have decided to buy a mandibular advancement device to move their jaw forward might need help with moulding it to fit. Many products need fine-tuning to suit the individual, and this is where we can help.

Anti-snoring remedies you can buy over the counter are broadly divided into two main types – sprays and mouthwashes, on the one hand, and gadgets of various types on the other. Some nasal decongestants, if used on a long-term basis, have been found to produce a condition called rhinitis medicamentosa, causing the nose lining to become cracked and dry, and sometimes even bleed. Rather than using a decongestant all the time, it might be worth while trying to find out why you are suffering from a permanently congested nose and getting treatment for the cause, not just the symptoms.

Here's a run-down on the products available at the time of writing.

Sprays and mouthwashes

Good Night Stop Snore mouthwash

This mouthwash, by Swiss Health, contains a selection of several different herbs and claims a 78-per-cent success rate in stopping snoring, as well as successful clinical trials. It is widely available from independent chemists. The *Health Which?* tester found he couldn't get the 'revolting' taste out of his mouth and was unwilling to persevere with the product. Swiss Health also produce the Good Night Stop Snore spray, described as 'a natural blend of oils that stimulates and tones the soft palate and clears sinus and bronchial mucus'. It contains vitamins C, B6 and E combined with natural oils, which include sunflower, peppermint, sesame and olive oil. It's available from independent pharmacies and health food stores.

Snoreeze throat spray

Snoreeze throat spray contains water, glycerine oil, peppermint oil and other oils, also vitamins B and E. The manufacturers claim 'instant snoring relief' if this is sprayed on the back of the throat, tongue and uvula. It is available from Superdrug, Holland & Barrett, Moss, GNC, independent pharmacies and health food stores. The *Health Which?* tester said it did seem to ease his breathing and snoring temporarily, even though he was still drinking alcohol. His partner, however, didn't notice any improvement.

Y-Snore nose drops

Y-Snore nose drops contain homeopathic tinctures of *Diosorea villosa* and *Zingiber officinale* and claim to 'relieve snoring fast'. They are available from the BSSAA. The *Health Which?* tester found that using the drops was unpleasant and left a bad taste in the mouth, but may have improved her snoring a little. The *Health Which?* experts were not terribly impressed with the quality of the research into this product.

Boots Alternative Snoring Remedy

This claims to 'help relieve snoring'. It contains eucalyptus oil, sage and thyme and should be sprayed on the back of the throat last thing at night. Boots claim that 82 per cent of patients using it report an improvement, but do not say how many patients were in their trial or whether or not the product is suitable for everyone including tongue-, nose- and palate-based snorers. This is a new product, not in the *Health Which?* tests, and is available only from Boots stores.

Helps Stop Snoring

Essential Health produce a spray and mouthwash called Helps Stop Snoring. This product was not included in the *Health Which?* survey but was tested on 140 couples by consultant ENT surgeon Andrew Pritchard. A reduction in snoring was reported by 82 per cent of the couples. Helps Stop Snoring is available from Boots, Sainsbury's, Waitrose, Morrisons and independent chemists.

Other herbal-type remedies

Companies that sell vitamins and health supplements by mail order also offer herbal-type snoring remedies.

Snore-Free

Woods Supplements of Luton sell Snore-Free, which they describe as a blend of natural oils and vitamins in a handy spray to aid instant snoring relief. Like most sprays, it's intended to coat the tissues at the back of the throat. For mail-order details call 0845 130 22 44.

Snorex

Another, similar product available by mail order is Snorex, described as a 'revolutionary new product made from natural ingredients in an advanced solution that allows oils to be dissipated throughout the night'. It is said to work by 'lubricating the tissue lining at the back of the throat including the tongue and soft palate'. The manufacturers claim that 'tests' have shown 'an incredible, immediate effect on reducing snoring in 9 out of 10 cases'. Snorex is available from Healthy Direct, St George's Place, St Peter Port, Guernsey GY1 3TT (tel. 0800 037 37 40) and comes with a 90-day money-back guarantee.

Snorestop

Health Which? also tested some tablets called Snorestop, bought

29

from an unspecified US website, that contain homoeopathic remedies. Their experts felt that results of clinical trials on this were interesting, but the tester thought the tablets took too long to dissolve and his partner reported little difference in his snoring patterns.

I Don't Snore spray

Health Aid's I Don't Snore spray is a nasal spray containing 'natural polysaccharides' that works by keeping the mucous membranes of the nose and the back of the throat moist and lubricated, so that they don't come into contact with one another and vibrate when air passes between them. For mail-order details on this product, phone 020 8426 3400. It's also available from independent chemists.

Never Snore

Higher Nature's Never Snore is available by mail order from Higher Nature, Burwash Common, East Sussex TN19 7LX. This product, which is GM-free and suitable for vegetarians and vegans, contains a 'unique combination of natural enzymes' that are said to metabolize the secretions at the back of the throat, together with herbs to reduce tissue swelling and open up the airway. The manufacturers report that Never Snore was tested on 220 subjects, 86 per cent of whom reported an improvement in their snoring, and that an independent study by *Good Housekeeping* magazine came up with similar results.

Gadgets

Breathe Right nasal strips

Stop snoring gadgets include Breathe Right nasal strips, which are similar in appearance to plasters. You stick them over the bridge of your nose and they claim to help keep congested nasal passages open. The *Health Which?* report made the point that although these strips seem to be well researched, only about 10 per cent of snoring is nose-based. Their tester found he could breathe more easily when using them, but still snored. As well as the 'regular' strips, there is a variant impregnated with Vick Vapor-Rub. Breathe Right strips are widely available from chemists and supermarkets.

The Nozovent

The Nozovent is a plastic gadget you wear in your nose, available in small, medium and large sizes, which is designed to dilate your nostrils and allow the air to flow freely. *Health Which?* experts felt that this could work, but again only for snorers whose problem was caused by blocked nostrils. Their tester found that the device made him feel constricted, and it later fell out. The Nozovent is available from the BSSAA.

The Somni Snore Guard

This is described as an 'oral vestibular shield', looks a bit like a gum shield and is worn in the mouth. It's designed to prevent mouth breathing and thus snoring. Like most of the products on sale it claims to be clinically tested, but on a fairly small number of snorers. The *Which?* experts pointed out that there would be a difference between having such a device properly fitted by a doctor or dentist and buying one over the counter. Their tester found it uncomfortable and obtrusive and said it didn't reduce snoring much. It is available from the BSSAA.

Mandibular advancement devices

More sophisticated and expensive gadgets are known as mandibular advancement devices, which work for tongue-based snorers by gently holding the lower jaw and tongue forward, giving you more space to breathe normally, and preventing the tongue falling backwards and blocking the airway. Although you can fit them yourself, the right fit is crucial and it would seem sensible to have an initial consultation with a dental expert before opting for this kind of treatment.

The Continuous Positive Airway Pressure machine

The ultimate gadget for intractable snorers and sufferers from sleep apnoea (see Chapter 7) is the Continuous Positive Airway Pressure, or CPAP, machine. This involves wearing a face mask attached to an air pump that lives beside the bed and blows carefully filtered air into the sleeper's airway all through the night, a bit like a reversed vacuum-cleaner. This is often seen as a treatment of last resort as, although effective, it's also expensive and can seem cumbersome. Machines, which need to be individually calibrated for each patient, can be very expensive, although prices in the UK are coming down all the time. You can't buy them in the shops as they are available on prescription only and normally after a sleep study has confirmed that this kind of treatment is appropriate. Sometimes CPAP machines are available on the NHS but it tends to depend, as with so many other treatments, on the budget of the individual NHS Trust. The machines are getting smaller and more sophisticated all the time, though NHS budgets mean the most basic models are most often prescribed. You can buy CPAP machines privately through the BSSAA.

The BSSAA catalogue

The BSSAA has a catalogue of anti-snoring remedies, including some of those in the *Health Which?* survey and others. Their catalogue does, helpfully, divide the remedies on offer into those suitable for different types of snorers. Among the products available from them are the Somni Snore Guard, Breathe Right nasal strips, Nozovent, Y-Snore and Snoreeze. They also list their own herbal spray, developed by a medical herbalist for use in the nasal passages and on the roof of the mouth, tightening these tissues and making it easier for the air to pass through. In addition, the BSSAA sells Ronfnyl, a herbal nasal spray from France. Both these are recommended for those with stuffy noses and catarrh.

Also in their catalogue are AirPlus Sleep nasal strips, which are similar to Breathe Right and are suitable for those whose snoring is caused by small or collapsing nostrils. There are two other gadgets for nose-based snorers, called Snore-No-More and NoseWide. The Snore-No-More is made of stainless steel and fits right up inside the nostrils, supporting the nasal cavity and preventing it from collapsing as you breathe in. NoseWide is a Swedish product consisting of two small hollow plastic plugs that you insert in each nostril to keep them clear.

Mouth breathers are catered for by the Chin-Up Strip. Described as a 'comfortable external support that helps to keep the mouth closed at night' it looks a bit like an oversized and chin-shaped sticking plaster.

For details of how to contact the BSSAA, see p. 83.

Consulting your GP

Most snorers will try at least some over-the-counter treatments before asking for help from their GP. As we noted earlier, if you had gone to your GP for help with a snoring problem 20 or 30 years ago you would probably have been told you had to live with it; but although GPs receive little training in the subject there is a lot more interest in possible help for snorers than there used to be. You will certainly be advised to lose weight, stop smoking and watch your alcohol intake. Lifestyle changes can do the trick in some cases (see Chapter 3).

BSSAA members report more sympathy from their doctors than was the case 10 or 20 years ago. Although some doctors are well informed about snoring issues – thanks, in part, to the efforts of organizations like the BSSAA who try to make sure that GP practices are targeted with their literature – not all are equally helpful.

'Problems usually arise when a GP doesn't know a great deal about the subject or where to refer someone for further help,' comments Marianne Davey of the BSSAA. 'Then the patient gets the feeling he doesn't care, which is usually not the case.'

Sleep studies

When self-help or simple remedies have failed to crack the problem, you can ask your GP to refer you to a sleep studies unit, a sleep clinic or possibly the ENT unit at your local hospital, depending on what is available in your area.

About 300 NHS hospitals have provision for sleep studies on-site, or home studies of sleep problems. In 1997, the BSSAA took a look at some of them and compared waiting times and facilities, which, as is often the case with the NHS, varied across the country. In about half a dozen units waiting time could be as little as two weeks, while in a few it was as long as six months.

'The impression we get is that waiting times may have increased as more patients need to be seen,' says Marianne Davey:

Hospitals and NHS Trusts only have so much money to go round and it has to be rationed, so we are finding that sleep clinics are beginning to be more strict about who they will see. Some will only see patients they suspect of having sleep apnoea, the most serious and dangerous form of snoring [see Chapter 7] but it does vary from area to area. A patient who is grossly overweight, smokes and drinks heavily and has high blood pressure will find it easier to get a sleep study than a younger, fitter person, who will probably be advised to make lifestyle changes first.

The aim of a sleep study is to find out exactly what is happening while the patient sleeps, and whether they are what Dr Peter Venn of the Sleep Studies Unit at the Queen Victoria Hospital in East Grinstead calls 'social snorers', or whether they suffer from some sort of breathing dysfunction that affects the quality of their sleep. This could include sleep apnoea (see Chapter 7), where the patient actually stops breathing for a few seconds at intervals during the night.

'It is important to distinguish between these two groups of patients, not least because their motivation is very different,' says Dr Venn:

> Patients in the second group will usually be suffering from sleep deprivation leading to extreme sleepiness and lethargy during the daytime, and the treatments offered will actually benefit them, as well as allowing their partners and families to get a good night's sleep.
>
> A sleep study involves the patient spending a night in the unit, attached to monitoring equipment which records information about their breathing patterns and transfers the information to a computer, a timed video and a microphone. We place a small nasal airflow sensor under the nose and the computer then records their breathing. They also need to wear a probe on their finger to measure the amount of oxygen in their blood. It's this lack of oxygen which leads to the health complications caused by dysfunctional breathing.
>
> If the study, called a 'polysomnogram', suggests that the patient does have a breathing problem, we will look at the video to see what is happening to the patient as their breathing patterns change. We can often tell whether the sound is coming from the soft palate or from behind the tongue. With the help of the video we can see whether the patient is lying on his back, gasping for air, or moving about in his sleep at this time. With all this information on hand we can usually tell what the problem is and whether we are dealing with a social snorer or someone with a more serious condition, and that has implications for the type of treatment. In my experience only about 3 to 5 per cent of patients will actually benefit from palatal surgery. For the others, a device which brings their jaw forward or a CPAP machine will be more appropriate.

Consulting your dentist

As well as doctors, dentists have also become involved in the treatment of snoring problems. The size and shape of the face and jaw help to determine whether someone will be a snorer or not. Most dental appliances are designed to pull the lower jaw and tongue forward to make more space at the back of the throat. Another kind of device can lift the soft palate to prevent vibration, or re-position the tongue. Specialist dentists will be able to advise you on which sort of appliance will suit you best, depending on the shape of your jaw and whether or not you still have all or most of your natural teeth. The British Dental Association experts say that properly positioned dental devices, which have to be individually made by specialist dental technicians, can reduce snoring. Dentists are now much better informed about sleep apnoea, the dangerous form of snoring, and often work with other medical experts in a multi-disciplinary approach to this problem.

Dr Joanna Battagel of the Department of Orthodontics at the Royal London Hospital emphasizes that the best way of obtaining this kind of treatment is after a referral from your GP to an ENT specialist or sleep studies unit has confirmed that you will benefit from it.

'It is important to obtain a correct diagnosis as dental devices are not appropriate for every snorer,' she says:

> There have been advertisements in the dental press suggesting that High Street dentists should be able to offer this kind of treatment direct to their patients, but it's safer to have a proper diagnosis. An overnight sleep study will confirm whether the patient is suffering from simple snoring or sleep apnoea. Tests will show where and how the airways are blocking. If the tongue is blocking the airway, a dental device may help, but it's important to be sure that you are not masking other problems like sleep apnoea, which can be serious and even life-threatening.

Dental devices

Dental devices to help snorers were pioneered in the USA some 20 years ago. 'There were a handful of American dentists working in the field at that time,' says Dr Battagel:

> Even today, they are not terribly common and High Street dentists

are only supposed to supply them after a prescription from a doctor or surgeon.

I know that you can buy over-the-counter dental devices from organizations like the BSSAA, and some patients do just that, often when they have grown tired of waiting to see a specialist. The BSSAA literature is very good and they will advise people, but I feel that off-the-shelf products have limitations. I have experimented with them and talked to patients about them. Buying one is rather like buying a sports mouth-guard. You dip them in hot water and mould them around your teeth for a good fit. However, I have found that they don't always bring the jaw far enough forward if you have a normal 'bite'. They can also be uncomfortable to wear, and they don't always stay in very well.

Dr Battagel explains that mandibular advancement devices are made of either hard or soft plastic and are designed to hold the lower jaw in an abnormally 'forward' position. Some are made in one piece and hold both top and bottom jaws in one position with very little freedom of movement. Others are in two pieces, allowing some movement.

'Some people feel rather claustrophobic if they can't move their jaw at all, and for them a two-piece device may be more comfortable,' she says:

It's rather like getting used to having a brace on your teeth, but on your lower and upper jaws.

I always explain to patients that there are likely to be some side-effects at first. Many people wake up with some muscular discomfort as the muscles they use to chew and their jaw joint may ache a little, but after about a week they will probably have got used to it. Some complain that the device makes them produce more saliva but others say it makes their mouth feel dry. It's a question of whether the discomfort or annoyance outweighs the advantages of not snoring. We did look at one group of patients after two years and found that about 60 to 70 per cent of them were still using their device. Often the ones who were using it because their snoring was disturbing other people gave up, while those who said that since using the device they were sleeping better and feeling more alert during the day were able to carry on.

Mandibular advancement devices don't suit all snorers, or even all tongue-based snorers. 'It's not easy to spot those who will be helped, which is why proper, expert diagnosis is important,' says Dr Battagel.

'There is such a wide range of facial shapes. People whose faces are flatter than average tend to benefit, and this includes people with small lower jaws whose tongues block the back of their throats.'

Less commonly used appliances are those that lift the soft palate to prevent vibration (which can make people gag) and those that are designed to hold the tongue forward by means of a type of suction, which can sometimes be used in patients who have no teeth of their own.

According to Dr Battagel, dental appliances are being refined all the time, and as this is a growing field more help may be available in future. In the USA, surgery is sometimes used to re-position both jaws but this is a drastic measure by British surgical standards. Few snorers, however desperate, would want to have both their jaws broken and then re-positioned, especially as this can alter the shape of the face and is, of course, a major operation that sometimes involves a spell in intensive care.

Mandibular advancement devices are not the only answer, says Dr Battagel:

> They won't work if a patient needs palatal surgery as well, or if this is someone who sleeps with their mouth very wide open. My advice would always be to have the snoring properly investigated by means of a sleep study before opting for this kind of treatment.

Buying a snoring remedy of any kind over the counter is always going to be a bit hit-and-miss. If you're absolutely certain your snoring is caused by a stuffy nose, then a nasal spray or decongestant of some kind, or a gadget designed to keep your nostrils open, may work for you.

The ingredients in throat sprays and mouthwashes vary but most are designed to lubricate the throat and firm up the floppy tissues. They do work – for some people. If you have tried two or three products to no effect, consult your GP or the BSSAA for the next step.

your snoring hasn't improved. It's a case of 'buyer beware'. The BSSAA is often approached by snorers who have had expensive surgery and found that it has made no difference to their snoring. They believe that as few as 1 per cent of snorers will actually benefit from surgery and found that, in a survey of 300 hospitals, only 6 actually undertook surgery as a remedy for snoring problems.

Some experts, too, remain unconvinced of the value of palatal surgery as a treatment for snoring. Dr Venn, of the Queen Victoria Hospital in East Grinstead, says that:

> The soft palate is there for a reason, to block your nose off when you swallow. Any form of surgery which removes part of the soft palate risks leaving the patient with a completely different set of problems. For instance, he might need to learn a new swallowing technique – a sort of gulp – or find that when he drinks a pint of beer it comes back down his nose because there's nothing left to stop it! Then there's the fact that palatal surgery is very painful and there is always a risk of infection. Some patients also say it leads to voice changes and more nasal speech, rather like a child with swollen adenoids.
>
> Laser surgery isn't without its problems either. Although it is intended to stiffen the palate with scar tissue, some patients find that their snoring comes back after a while. Nasal surgery can sometimes work if the patient has a genuine problem with a permanently blocked nose, but lifestyle changes and/or a CPAP machine still represent the gold standard of treatment for most patients.

It might sound unfair if your doctor tells you to go away and lose weight before he considers an operation, but he is not just being mean. Surgery produces better results on thin snorers than fat ones – it's as simple as that.

Who can benefit?

Selecting the right patients to benefit from surgery is a co-operative venture, often involving both physicians and surgeons and a sleep studies unit.

'GPs should be able to tell patients about the most common reasons for snoring, like being overweight or drinking too much or having a stuffy nose because of hay fever,' says Grant Bates, consultant ENT surgeon at the Radcliffe Infirmary in Oxford:

> When a patient is referred to an ENT specialist we first have to find out, often with the help of their partner, whether their problem is severe snoring or if there are features which suggest sleep apnoea, such as excessive daytime sleepiness, restless sleep and breath-holding episodes.
>
> Sometimes the reasons for the snoring are simple. An obstruction in the upper airway might require steroids to be prescribed, or if there is a bent septum – the bit between the nostrils – a straightforward nasal operation could alleviate the problem.
>
> I use a flexible, very thin fibre-optic telescope to look at the back of the nose and see how long the soft palate is, and if there is any redundant tissue. This examination can be done in the outpatients department with a local anaesthetic to numb the nose, and it's quite painless. If a sleep study shows that there is no sleep apnoea and the patient is 'just' a bad snorer, and simple cures have been tried and have not worked, then UPPP could be the treatment of choice. It is the most painful ENT operation, though, so no one should have it if it's not absolutely necessary. With correctly selected patients, it has an 80-per-cent success rate in curing snoring. Patients for whom it doesn't work are usually those who have additional problem features as well as a floppy soft palate and large tonsils – for example, an especially fat neck, a crowded mouth and a receding chin.

UPPP surgery actually involves removing a section of the palate and the tonsils, especially if they are very large, and is carefully tailored to the individual patient. Grant Bates says that British surgeons are pretty conservative about the amount of tissue they remove:

> If you take away too much, there's a possibility of food going up the nose afterwards, when the patient begins to eat. I feel it's better to leave someone snoring slightly than with post-operative speech problems or other long-term side-effects. If the tonsils are very large, simply removing them might cure the problem.
>
> The operation lasts about half an hour and usually involves a one-night stay in hospital. I always tell my patients to expect some pain for about ten days afterwards. There will be a raw area at the back of the throat where there are a lot of nerve endings.

Mr Bates says that using a laser to perform surgery makes little difference in this respect; in fact, laser surgery can be even more painful as it actually burns the tissue at a high temperature, unlike the harmonic scalpel used in UPPP that melts the tissue at only 50 degrees.

Like all ENT experts, he reminds his patients that if their weight increases, snoring problems may return. 'With obesity increasing among the general population we are going to see more snorers,' he says:

But people are trying new methods all the time. In the USA more complicated and invasive surgery is used and there have been other innovations, like a paste which was used to stiffen the soft palate in some patients. A surgeon in Cambridge did try that but although he had a good success rate at first, in the longer term it was found that many patients continued to snore.

Surgery does work for some people but the message, even from surgeons, is that snorers should try to lose weight and cut down on their alcohol consumption.

Successful surgery: Ken and Hugh and UPPP

Ken and Hugh are both ex-snorers for whom surgery – UPPP in both cases – was successful.

'My snoring woke me in the night occasionally, and I never slept really well,' says Ken:

It was much more of a problem for my wife! She suffers from rheumatoid arthritis and sleeps badly anyway so she encouraged me to seek treatment. I must have tried every possible off-the-shelf remedy but, quite honestly, found them all a waste of time and money. I tried sprays, mouthwashes, gadgets meant to widen my nostrils, plaster strips I wore across my nose, even sticky tape across my mouth, but my wife said I was still a violent snorer.

My GP was very sympathetic and referred me to my local ENT department. As I had tried all the normal remedies, I don't smoke or drink and am about the right weight, I was told I would be suitable for surgery. I had to fill in a form to see if I had the symptoms of sleep apnoea, but I didn't.

I was told the operation would be painful but in the event I found it more uncomfortable, and I was given painkillers anyway. I had to stay in hospital overnight and it was all very straightforward. My tonsils were not removed, and unfortunately some time after the operation I picked up an infection that made them swell up and narrow the airway in my throat, so although the violent snoring has stopped I am still not a quiet sleeper. However, I have been treated with antibiotics and the problem is improving. Both my wife and I can now get a good night's sleep.

Hugh describes his UPPP surgery as the best thing he ever did, after struggling for 15 years with a severe snoring problem:

It became so bad that my wife and I didn't sleep together any more. Holidays were difficult when my children were younger because they couldn't share a family room with us. Once my son ended up sleeping on the hotel balcony. Sharing a room with a colleague on a business trip was out of the question. I even had fellow-guests knocking on the walls of my hotel room begging me to keep the noise down. I tried all the old wives' remedies, like sewing a tennis ball in the back of my pyjamas, and cut down on smoking and drinking. My wife became so desperate that she bought me all kinds of throat sprays and mouthwashes, but nothing worked.

Seven years ago, we were divorced, though not because of my snoring. After a couple of years apart we got back together again, and by that time my snoring was so bad that my wife said I really had to have something done about it. I had heard about operations you could have using a laser and actually enquired about the possibility, but then I heard about someone who had died after the operation, which put me off. When we re-married I went back to my GP who referred me to an ENT surgeon. A year later I had the operation. I can't praise the hospital enough. I had to go in before the operation for 24-hour monitoring to measure my heart rate, and the nurse explained to me exactly what the operation would involve.

Unfortunately I had a haemorrhage in the recovery room and had to go back into theatre. I went home the next day but had a couple more haemorrhages and then picked up some kind of infection. I was ill for about three weeks in all, but, to me, that was a small price to pay. I was told that my tonsils were very large so they were removed together with a lot of floppy tissue. The result was a 200-per-cent improvement, not only in my snoring but in the quality of my life generally. I no longer smoke. I sleep through the night without waking up, I don't feel tired during the day, and my wife and I have a normal married life again. She used to say my snoring made the windows rattle until she felt like killing me. Snorers' partners and families have a lot to put up with!

Coblation

'I won't operate on people with a BMI of more than 25,' says consultant ENT surgeon Mike Timms of the Abbey Gisburne Park Hospital in Gisburn, Lancashire, who uses the new coblation technique on his patients. 'Three-quarters of the people referred to me are overweight. If they lost weight, they probably would not need surgery at all.'

Mr Timms first used coblation on his young tonsillectomy patients and found the technique resulted in much less post-operative pain than conventional surgery. He is currently using the same technique to treat snorers.

'Like many surgeons performing this kind of operation, I wanted to find a less painful but equally effective method,' he explains:

There are two ways of using coblation. One is a minimalist approach, under local anaesthetic, probing the soft palate. This works for some people but I didn't find it radical enough and I was only getting a 50-per-cent response. The other method is basically UPPP, but using this instrument instead of a scalpel, which causes less pain and achieves an equal success rate. I use an 'Evac 70' handpiece, the same as I use for tonsillectomies, and I have found that patients are in much less pain afterwards. They can eat, as well. It works because it is a much cooler process. Coblation operates at 60 degrees, compared with the 300 degrees plus for lasers and the same for conventional diathermy. The instrument I use is saline irrigated and with inbuilt suction, which has advantages. From the surgeon's point of view, there's hardly any blood, so we don't have to cauterize surrounding areas to stem bleeding – and the result is much less pain for the patient.

However, Mr Timms stresses that the important factor in the success of any anti-snoring surgery is selecting the right patients. There is no point in operating on the palate if the problem lies elsewhere. It is possible that a tongue-based snorer could undergo major maxillo-facial surgery to realign the jaw, but again this would be a treatment of last resort. One of the mandibular advancement devices that can be fitted inside the mouth by a dentist might be a better solution.

He explains that appropriate surgery is available for people with nasal problems too:

> Someone with a bent septum, enlarged turbinates (the side bones in the nose) or nasal polyps, once diagnosed, can be treated too. A septum can be straightened, turbinates could be trimmed or shrunk by means of a laser, coblation if appropriate, diathermy or freezing, and polyps could be removed by an intranasal polypectomy.

LAUP

Andrew Birzgalis of the BUPA Manchester Hospital has been treating snorers for 20 years using laser palatoplasty on those patients who will benefit from it. 'When people come for an initial diagnosis I generally recommend that they lose weight – although I rarely see patients who are very overweight as they will not be referred to me because they will not be suitable for surgery,' he says:

> We then have to find out exactly where their snoring is coming from. Some people will need to take home a small portable monitor which enables us to review their snoring. The soft palate is the most common source and most surgery concentrates on that area. Whether you stiffen up the soft tissue with laser treatments, freeze it or microwave it, the effect is that scarring of the soft tissue tightens it up so that it doesn't flap and make a noise when air is breathed in past it. It is sometimes possible to tell where a patient's snoring originates by listening to the sound they make. Palate-based snorers make a flapping sound, unlike the constant sound made by tongue-based snorers.
>
> I use a laser because it doesn't require a general anaesthetic and it is less traumatic to the tissues. Basically you are just burning off the floppy bits, and like most surgeons I want to find the least traumatic way of doing the job. Patients can expect their throats

to be painful for seven to ten days after surgery, however the operation is carried out.

Some patients who opt for laser surgery find that they need as many as four to six sessions before there is a real impact on their snoring, but Mr Birzgalis says this is not always true: 'Most of my patients see a difference after just one session,' he says.

There is a small percentage for whom the operation doesn't work. This may be because their snoring is tongue-based or because it is coming from somewhere deeper in their throat. The other point to make is that it's important, after surgery, to carry on following a healthy lifestyle and keeping your weight down, or the snoring is likely to recur.

I did carry out a follow-up study on some of my patients and about 40 per cent said they had had some recurrence of their snoring between two and five years later. In about 20 per cent of cases, this was quite significant. However, it is quite difficult to measure how much worse or better snoring has become over a period of time. Surgery for snoring is not an exact science, but most patients seem very happy with the results.

Whatever the final choice of operation, getting the diagnosis right is the first step. No one should consider surgery until a sleep study has shown that they could benefit from it. If you and your doctors do decide it's the best treatment for you, you should make sure that they give you a good idea of what the operation will involve, what the side-effects might be – and what the chances are of your snoring returning at a later date.

6

Complementary Medicine

More and more of us are using complementary therapies for our day-to-day healthcare. Sometimes this is because of frustration with the limitations of conventional medicine and sometimes it's because we feel it's a more natural approach without the side-effects of prescription drugs. There's no doubt that complementary medicines can be effective in treating some common ailments. But do they have anything to offer the snorer?

Over-the-counter cures

Several of the over-the-counter 'snoring cures' already mentioned in Chapter 4 are actually based on the principles of complementary medicine. Most include herbal ingredients and essential oils, and some snorers do seem to find the sprays, mouthwashes and gargles helpful in controlling their snoring. As with other remedies, though, it does depend on *why* you snore. If you suffer from nasal congestion, sinus problems or an allergy, herbal preparations can sometimes be useful. Most claim to work by toning up the loose, floppy tissues at the back of the throat, and if this is your problem, you might find they work for you.

Boots Alternative Snoring Remedy, for example, comes in the form of a spray and contains eucalyptus oil, which has anti-bacterial properties, thyme, which has antiseptic properties, and sage 'for clearing the head'. Snoreeze, which is described as a 'unique throat spray made from natural oils and vitamins' actually contains water, glycerine, olive oil, peppermint oil, soya lecithin, sunflower seed oil, sweet almond oil, sesame oil and vitamins E and B6. Snoreeze is designed to coat the soft tissues in the throat that vibrate to cause snoring. A research study in 2000 found the product to be effective in reducing snoring noise, but involved only 28 couples.

'Men sometimes find it hard to admit to personal problems, even though there must be thousands of snorers out there,' says 58-year-old John, a snorer for 20 years:

I thought that my weight might be a factor, and also my build, as I

47

have quite a thick neck. I had never even been to my GP. I'm not sure why not, except that I was afraid he would suggest an operation. I know someone who paid £1,000 for surgery at a Harley Street clinic. The operation didn't work and I didn't want to waste my money.

Snoring caused me huge problems. We used to live in a flat and I was so embarrassed when my downstairs neighbour told me she had had to move into her back bedroom because my snoring was keeping her awake – so you can imagine how loud it was! My wife spent most nights in our spare room. She did tape me snoring once and I couldn't believe the noise I made.

We adopted a dog from a rescue centre and she was very nervous of any loud noises. When we took her to an animal behaviourist he told us that my snoring was probably at the root of her problems too.

I tried those plaster strips that athletes wear. They helped for a time, but not for long. I tried a nasal spray and a sort of plastic gadget but none of them were very effective. Then I tried Snoreeze. The difference with this product is you spray it on the back of your throat and it firms up the muscles there. The difference was amazing. My snoring stopped virtually straight away. It was great for me and my wife. We now sleep together after years apart and we both get a good night's sleep – and so does our dog!

Dahm's Goodnight, by Swiss Health, is a widely available blend of essential oils, including rosemary, sage, lavender, peppermint and fennel, combined with the active ingredient mastic oil, which, it's claimed, gently tones the muscles and increases blood flow so that the tissues are less likely to vibrate. You can buy it in the form of a spray or a mouthwash, and it's basically a herbal product that has been subjected to clinical trials in Germany and Russia.

'We were sceptical about trying a natural remedy, having tried nose plasters and even considered surgery as the noise was horrendous,' says one user's wife. 'But the effects were almost immediate. The snoring noise reduced after the first night, and eventually stopped completely after a couple of nights, making us both a lot happier!'

'Alternative' practitioners

Would it help to consult an 'alternative' practitioner? I contacted representatives of the most frequently used complementary therapies and asked them what they could offer snorers. The first piece of advice they gave was to make sure, when you are thinking of trying any complementary medicine or therapy, that the person you consult is properly qualified and a member of a recognized professional organization (addresses on pp. 84–86).

Herbal medicine

Traditional plant remedies still provide about 85 per cent of the world's medicines. Herbalism is part of a long tradition stretching back thousands of years and many of the drugs we use today, from aspirin to certain anti-cancer drugs, were originally derived from plant sources. Medical herbalists are trained to treat the patient as a whole – holistically – rather than looking at individual symptoms.

'If someone came to me with a snoring problem I would first look at their general health and how long the problem had been going on,' says Trudy Norris of the National Institute of Medical Herbalists:

> I might suggest that the patient adjusted their diet and/or life-style – perhaps reducing or eliminating dairy products from the diet. Certainly, snoring that was caused by sinus or allergy problems would be amenable to herbal treatment. For a sinus problem I would use those herbs which can affect excess mucus production. If the problem stemmed from an allergy I would look at other ways in which the allergy manifested itself and possibly treat with herbs which can ameliorate an over-active immune response. Another possibility would be to use herbs to tonify the mucous membranes in the throat.
>
> There might also be a structural element involved, for instance misaligned cranial vertebrae, for which manipulation might be prescribed. I would then suggest that the patient come back in two weeks, and again in a month, by which time something should be happening. Snoring is a chronic problem so it's unlikely to stop overnight, but there are several things a herbalist could suggest which might help.

Homoeopathy

Another well-established complementary therapy, homoeopathy is based on the principle that 'like cures like'. Illnesses are treated with minute doses of substances that, when taken by a healthy person, would produce symptoms similar to those displayed by the sick person. It is thought to work by stimulating the body's natural forces of recovery and concentrates on treating the patient, not the disease.

Registered homoeopath Sara Rossi says:

> Snoring is certainly not a joke. I have heard of people whose relationships are destroyed by one partner's snoring. Over-the-counter homoeopathic medicines can be useful but you would get better results from a consultation.
>
> The point about homoeopathy is that it is individual and symptom-orientated. I would always take a full case history, including asking when the patient first became aware of the problem, because people are often unaware that they snore. It could be caused by an allergic reaction to pollution in the home or outside; it could be the result of blocked sinuses with all the implications that has for liver or kidney pathology. It could be diet-related – dairy products and oranges are foods which produce excess mucus in some people. It could even be a physical or emotional reaction to the person the patient is sleeping with. Once they are given a safe arena in which to talk, many things are revealed. Snoring is normally a concomitant of something else; there are other things going on in the body. Homoeopathy offers more than 3,000 possible remedies to choose from, and it's not just about selecting the right remedy – it's also about the potency and the dosage, when and how the remedy or combination of remedies is prescribed. But without any doubt, homoeopathy can help.

Sara is also a qualified yoga teacher and says that yoga, with its emphasis on breathing, as well as learning specific breathing techniques, can help snorers too.

Traditional Chinese medicine (TCM)

TCM has been developed over the past 4,000 years and, if anything, the Chinese regard Western medicine as the 'alternative'! TCM is based on totally different principles from Western medicine and believes in treating the underlying cause of any medical problem, rather than the symptoms, as in Western medicine. Chinese doctors believe that almost all medical problems are the result of an imbalance of the body's internal systems, and will treat their patients accordingly, often with a combination of special Chinese herbs and acupuncture.

'Snoring is not a simple matter,' says Professor Man Fong Mei of the Acumedic Centre in London:

It could be caused by many syndromes, including muscle block, which is governed by the spleen, or an energetic block, which is governed by the liver. Obviously it can also involve the lungs. A Chinese physician would make an individual diagnosis and prescribe treatment tailored to that individual. Some patients may require an operation and Chinese medicine is very helpful when a patient is recovering after surgery.

Ayurvedic medicine

Like traditional Chinese medicine, Ayurvedic medicine has a long and distinguished history, having been practised in India for more than 3,000 years. It is based on the principle that there are three forces or vital energies, known as *doshas*, and that an imbalance in these leads to health disorders. The three *doshas* are called *vata*, *pitta* and *kapha*, and good health requires balancing these doshas within the body. Practitioners say that people who are *kapha* types (large-boned, overweight, pale-complexioned and slow-moving, with calm personalities) are most prone to snoring and other respiratory disorders.

According to Dr Moorthy of the Ayurvedic Medical Association UK, treatment for snoring will be tailored to the individual patient and will include cleansing therapy, involving steam inhalation, oil to put into the nose, and gargling, plus breathing exercises to clear the nasal passages and throat. Herbal medicines are also sometimes prescribed. Ayurvedic medicine recognizes that snoring is a symptom and will look for the causes, for instance excess mucus production or smoking, before prescribing. Lifestyle and dietary changes may also be recommended.

Hypnotherapy

Hypnotherapy is often misunderstood. It's not about being out of control, or about being made to do something you wouldn't otherwise do. A properly qualified hypnotherapist will induce a state of relaxed awareness in her patient, a state that has sometimes been compared with daydreaming. Once in that state, the subconscious is much more receptive to suggestion. Hypnotherapy can be used to help both snorers and, more particularly, their partners.

Maggie Chapman is a hypnotherapist, and a member of the British Society of Clinical Hypnosis, who has successfully treated both snorers and partners. She maintains that any treatment must be combined with lifestyle changes and that the snorer must be motivated to change. 'If the motivation is not there, I will ask to treat the partner instead,' she says:

> Snoring can cause huge problems in relationships, especially if the partner feels the snorer is not prepared to give up their brandy-and-cigars lifestyle.
>
> If someone is overweight and drinking heavily, hypnotherapy can help them to make the necessary lifestyle changes. Then I would also use simple, direct suggestion to 'lighten' the sleep so that the snorer could hear himself snore, turn over, perhaps change position and go back to sleep again. Normally, snorers are so deeply asleep that they can't hear themselves – although their unconscious can!
>
> If I was working with a snorer's partner who was suffering the misery of sleep deprivation, I would help them to sleep more deeply by re-framing the noise or showing them how to experience it as soothing, like a cat's purr, rather than irritating. The way hypnotherapy works is to access a deep state of relaxation and then install these suggestions.

Bach Flower Remedies

Dr Edward Bach, a Harley Street physician and homoeopath, noticed that patients suffering from emotional problems benefited from the same homoeopathic remedy, whatever their physical symptoms. He devised a series of plant-based remedies to treat a total of 38 negative or harmful states of mind. According to a spokesman at the Bach Centre in Oxfordshire, Bach Flower Remedies may possibly benefit both the snorer and his or her partner:

> Three possibilities come to mind. Bach remedies are used to treat emotional states, so if there are lifestyle factors that aggravate someone's snoring problem – alcohol abuse, for example – a remedy might help to deal with the reasons why the person is engaging in that behaviour.
>
> Also, the snorer's partner might be helped. There are a number of remedies effective in dealing with the emotions roused by snoring, like irritation, anger or self-pity. If the partner was angry,

beech might be selected. If they were unable to sleep because of the snoring, then I might select walnut, which is for outside influences which affect the emotional state. Having said that, it wouldn't make the snoring go away!

Or, if the snorer felt guilty about the problems he or she was causing, pine might be useful in dealing with that.

Bach remedies might be used to treat the emotions aroused by the snoring, rather than the snoring itself.

Acupuncture

Acupuncture works by inserting fine needles into the body to stimulate the invisible 'meridians' – lines of energy that run beneath the surface of the skin – to balance the body's energy and encourage the body to heal itself. Acupuncture has been in use in the Far East, India and South-East Asia for over 2,000 years and is becoming an increasingly popular therapy in the West since it can be used alongside Western medicine.

Like other complementary practitioners, acupuncturist Hilary Coles, who practises in Yorkshire and is also a tutor at the Northern College of Acupuncture in York, says that it's vitally important to make sure anyone you consult is registered with the British Acupuncture Council.

'Acupuncture can be used to treat general respiratory problems including snoring,' she says:

> Some people don't respond, as with any therapy, but others do. If a snorer consulted me I would first take a history and decide which energy seemed to be disturbed in which organ. Perhaps the patient's lungs are low in *chi* – the flow of vital energy – or there may be an imbalance in the large intestine channel which runs past the nose. Once the diagnosis was made I would formulate a point prescription and insert the needles around the body at the appropriate points.
>
> Snoring is a serious problem, affecting not only the patient but the people around him, too, and I would say that acupuncture treatment is worth a try.

Acupressure, or 'acupuncture without needles', which involves applying pressure to the appropriate points on the body to unblock vital energy, works in a similar way. You can be taught to apply pressure to the right points yourself.

Alexander Technique

Frederick Matthias Alexander was an Australian actor, famous for his one-man Shakespeare recitals. He lost his voice and regained it only after studying his posture, which led to him devising his method of helping people to achieve balance and poise with minimal muscle tension. The technique is often practised by actors and singers to improve breathing and voice projection. Alexander teachers believe that it is not possible to separate health problems – including snoring – from what is going on in the rest of the body, especially the spine.

The Alexander Technique is preventative and aims to restore a better balance so that a pupil will experience the body moving freely, as it should. However, it's not just about posture and relaxation, but about self-improvement and self-help.

Alexander teacher Marjorie Hodge says that there is no official research proving that the technique can help snoring, but that there is some anecdotal evidence and that pupils do find it beneficial.

Reiki

Reiki is a form of energy healing, involving a gentle, hands-on technique that uses universal energy to enhance physical and mental well-being. As with many complementary therapies it is very much tailored to the individual and concentrates on accelerating the healing process, bringing peace and balance. The word *reiki* is Japanese and means Universal–Life–Force–Energy. A 'cure' is not guaranteed but Reiki can have a calming effect on both snorers and their partners.

Yoga

Breathing exercises are a fundamental part of yoga. If your snoring is caused by nasal congestion, then practising yoga could help to keep your airways open. A spokeswoman for the British Wheel of Yoga says that a combination of correct breathing, cleansing techniques and attention to diet resulting in weight loss can have a marked effect on snoring.

'The first thing is to clear the nasal passages,' she says:

A saline solution called *jala neti* is poured through the nostrils to clear them of excess mucus. Once the nostrils are cleared, breathing exercises can begin. A particularly effective one is known as *bramari rama* or 'the bee' because that is what it sounds like. It is rather like humming and reverberates in the nose, but the lips also vibrate, which helps to clear the nostrils.

Diet is also very important. Quite often people who produce too much mucus are eating too many dairy products. If you cut down on these the problem may disappear.

If, when someone lies down and tries to relax when practising yoga, they are inclined to snore, we put something under the head, or put them in the recovery position. We also advise them to keep their chin down, because when the chin goes up the mouth tends to open and then you get snoring.

Any yoga teacher should be able to advise someone who is concerned about snoring and help them to keep their airways clear.

Magnet therapy

Using magnets for healing has a long history. Magnet therapy was known to the ancient Greeks, Chinese and Egyptians – Cleopatra is said to have worn magnets to maintain her legendary beauty! Modern-day magnet therapy is popular in Eastern Europe and Japan, where magnetic wrist bands and other products are used to treat many conditions, particularly bone disorders like osteoporosis, and also fractures. Conventional medicine uses electrical equipment to generate electro-magnetic fields that influence the body's natural electric currents and promote healing. Magnet therapists believe that a magnet placed on the body can enhance blood flow and improve the supply of oxygen, stimulate the metabolism and help to eliminate waste. A company called Magnetic Therapy, based in Manchester, sells a range of magnetic products including the Snore-Free, a small plastic ring containing two rare earth magnets, developed by an ex-NASA scientist. The ring is attached to the nose, stimulating the sensory nerves and opening the nasal passages, helping to prevent snoring. If your snoring is caused by nasal congestion this could be one to try. The Snore-Free is available by mail order from Freephone 0845 130 5110, or can be ordered online from www.magnetictherapy.co.uk.

A combination of techniques

Some complementary practitioners find that a combination of techniques can be helpful in dealing with common medical problems, including snoring. Dr Mosaraf Ali, of the Integrated

Medical Centre in London, recommends a programme that incorporates lifestyle changes with the use of essential oils, Ayurvedic medicine and yoga. His suggestions include:

- a diet rich in fruit and vegetables, organic if possible, and avoiding coffee, yeast-containing foods, sugar, excess alcohol, rich and spicy food;
- fresh air and daily exercise;
- an early evening meal followed by a 15-minute walk;
- five minutes of yoga before bed, particularly the Cobra, Semi-bridge and Turtle poses;
- breathing stale air, containing less oxygen and more carbon dioxide, by covering your nose lightly with a sheet or duvet;
- making sure you're not overheated by using lightweight bedding and ensuring the bedroom is well ventilated;
- the use of Dr Ali's massage oil or sinus oil and/or the Ayurvedic supplement Mentat (for mail-order details on these products see p. 86).

At the Hale Clinic in London, a variety of complementary therapies are on offer. Duja Purkit, a therapist there, has had considerable success in treating snoring using a combination of dietary changes, Indian massage and essential oils.

'Snoring is often caused by an excess of mucus in the nose and throat which produces a breathing block,' he says:

> My aim in treatment is to reduce the amount of mucus. I look at the patient's diet and cut out mucus-producing foods like dairy produce and fried food. Then I place two drops of sesame oil in each nostril and begin to massage between the eyebrows and on both cheeks, for two minutes on each side. I then give the patient breathing exercises – breathing in for a count of two and out for a count of three. Occasionally herbal tablets are also necessary.
>
> Dryness of the nose area can also cause snoring. If this is the case I treat the patient with two or three drops of good-quality, alcohol-free rosewater in each nostril. Dryness can also be caused by liver problems so I try to find a way to improve the patient's liver function. Papaya after breakfast is very good for the liver. When the condition improves the dryness is reduced and the patient is able to breathe in quietly.
>
> Treatments for snoring are always tailored to the individual. I

find when children have a snoring problem, an effective treatment is to warm sesame oil with a clove of garlic and rub it on the child's chest. This has a powerful warming effect and the child's lung function improves.

Aisha's young son began receiving Indian massage treatment at the Hale Clinic when he was two years old:

> He was always a snuffly baby who snored when he was asleep and breathed heavily through his mouth when he was awake. He just didn't seem able to breathe through his nose and had hearing problems. He had grommets inserted at the hospital but they didn't help his breathing. We took him to Duja who would massage him using oils, around his shoulders, his neck, and on his forehead and temples. Within about ten minutes of the massage starting my son would be asleep and his breathing became quieter and clearer. I was so impressed that I took a cousin who suffered from very bad nasal congestion due to hay fever, and massage seemed to help him as well.

If you're a sceptic about 'alternative' therapies, you probably won't want to consider using them to help with your snoring problem. There are few placebo-controlled, double-blind clinical trials written up in reputable medical journals that 'prove', once and for all, that homoeopathy, yoga or traditional Chinese medicine guarantees a cure, especially for a problem like snoring that can have a variety of causes.

On the other hand, reputable complementary therapists have many years of experience and a long tradition of working holistically to help patients with every kind of medical condition. It's worth remembering that the majority of over-the-counter snoring remedies are pretty much based on herbs and similar ingredients. If your snoring seems to be the result of nasal congestion – or you're the long-suffering partner of a snorer – you may find a consultation with a complementary practitioner worth while.

7

Sleep Apnoea

Snoring, as we've already established, is not funny, either for the snorer or for those who live with him. It can be exasperating, maddening and frustrating. However, it's not, in itself, normally a danger to health – except in the sense that some of the causes of snoring, like being overweight and drinking to excess, can lead to more serious health problems as well.

There is one type of snoring that *is* actually dangerous. It's known as sleep apnoea. The word 'apnoea' comes from a Greek word meaning 'want of breath', and sleep apnoea happens when no air at all passes through the nose or mouth for up to ten seconds at a time. In other words, the sleeper temporarily stops breathing. About 2 per cent of all sleepers are said to suffer from sleep apnoea, and many remain undiagnosed, which has implications not only for their physical and mental health but for public safety, if they are drivers or in charge of machinery. According to the Sleep Apnoea Trust, the support group for sufferers that is based in High Wycombe, about 80,000 people in Britain suffer from the condition. Most (but not all) are men, most (but not all) are overweight, especially around the neck, and they all snore.

Types of sleep apnoea

There are three types of sleep apnoea. The most common is **obstructive sleep apnoea** (OSA).

We have already learned that snoring is caused by the airways at the back of the throat narrowing and the breathed-in air making a noise as it hits the floppy, relaxed tissues. In cases of obstructive sleep apnoea, the airway 'falls in on itself' and becomes completely blocked. Partial obstruction of the airway (causing snoring) is replaced by total obstruction (causing sleep apnoea). The sleeper is often unaware of what is happening. If his partner is awake to see it, it can appear quite frightening, as he may seem to choke and gasp for air before resuming normal breathing. Fortunately, the body is able to sense that the brain is being deprived of oxygen in this way and a safety mechanism kicks in, waking the sleeper very briefly to take a gasp of air and then begin breathing again. Someone with severe sleep apnoea will experience a continuous cycle of blocked airways, gasping and choking and sudden awakenings, often as frequently as a hundred times a night.

Central sleep apnoea (CSA) happens when the brain doesn't send the right signals to tell you to breathe when you are asleep, and **mixed sleep apnoea** (MSA) is a mixture of OSA and CSA.

In order to benefit from a really good night's sleep, and awake refreshed and restored, we have to get *enough* sleep, although individual needs vary. Lady Thatcher is someone who apparently has always needed little sleep, as were Napoleon and Winston Churchill, whereas Albert Einstein needed a lot. *Quality* of sleep matters just as much as quantity, though, and quality sleep is just what people with sleep apnoea don't get. Sound sleepers go through several sleep cycles in the night. The development of the EEG – electroencephalogram – machine has enabled sleep researchers to discover just what happens to the brain and body during sleep and to identify the different stages of sleep, characterized by different brain-wave patterns.

Drowsiness, sometimes known as stage one sleep, leads on to deeper and deeper levels of sleep, each with its own characteristic brain waves. In stage four sleep, the deepest level, brain waves are much larger and slower. It's in this deep sleep that blood cells and body tissues are rebuilt and energy levels are restored. In an average night, a sound sleeper will also experience from one to two hours of rapid eye movement (REM) or 'dreaming' sleep. During REM sleep there are physiological changes including irregular breathing and heartbeat, increased blood flow and fluctuating blood pressure.

We sleep in cycles of roughly 90 to 100 minutes, passing through sleep stages one to four, then going back to stage two, then into a REM phase. The precise function of the cycles of non-REM and REM sleep we go through is not yet known, but both kinds of sleep are known to be vital for healthy physical and mental functioning. People with sleep apnoea don't get a chance to experience the benefits of really deep sleep. Because they keep waking, or semi-waking, they remain 'stuck' in the early, lighter sleep stages. Sleep apnoea can be at its worst during REM sleep, when the muscles are so relaxed that it takes longer than usual for the body to respond to the signals the brain is sending about oxygen deprivation. This may be the reason why sufferers can develop memory and intellect problems, as well as other symptoms like extreme sleepiness, mood changes and loss of libido.

Not surprisingly, sleep apnoea sufferers never get a good night's sleep, although they may not realize what is causing the problem. They will probably suffer from severe daytime sleepiness with all the problems that causes, including irritability and lack of concentration as well as a habit of falling asleep at inappropriate times. According to the British Lung Foundation, people with sleep apnoea are about seven times more likely to have car accidents than the rest of us. About 10 per cent of all accidents are caused by driver fatigue, and although it is not known how big a part sleep apnoea plays in these, it would seem likely that it is a contributory factor. Sleep-related accidents have a high mortality rate and it's estimated that every fatal road accident costs the country over £800,000. As it only costs about £250 to treat the average sleep apnoea sufferer, it has been estimated that 3,200 patients could be treated for the cost of a single fatal road crash.

Recently there have been several high-profile cases of drivers falling asleep at the wheel and causing horrific crashes, including the Selby train crash and an accident on the motorway in Kent. In that case, a lorry driver who was a sleep apnoea sufferer smashed his vehicle into an oncoming car, killing its occupants. Sleep studies units are accustomed to treating patients who work as bus- and lorry-drivers, with all the safety implications that has for the rest of us.

Poor-quality sleep and daytime tiredness is a much bigger problem than is often realized. With hospitals often forced to compete for resources, one expert pointed out that it is considerably cheaper to treat someone for sleep apnoea than it is to treat the same person, later, for a heart attack or stroke, not to mention the additional cost of treating the road-accident victims of tired drivers! The Head of Road Safety at the Royal Society for the Prevention of Accidents makes the point that driving while sleepy is stupid and selfish. His message is a blunt one: if you are tired, stay off the road. This means that if you are a sleep apnoea sufferer, you are not a safe driver until your condition has been diagnosed and treated. Don't take chances with your life, or anyone else's.

The BSSAA say that UK doctors have been slow even to recognize the condition. Unfortunately, some people going to their GPs complaining of poor sleep and reduced quality of life have been prescribed anti-depressants, which can make sleep apnoea worse. Others have been diagnosed with high blood pressure and prescribed beta-blockers, which, again, can make sleep apnoea worse. According to Professor Neil Douglas of Edinburgh University, only around

1 in 20 patients with the syndrome are so far being diagnosed and treated.

More awareness of the problem among the medical profession means that things are improving and that it shouldn't be too difficult to obtain a diagnosis and more appropriate treatment today.

Quite apart from the dangers posed by being continually tired, sleep apnoea can lead to other health problems. Severe morning headaches, depression and personality changes have all been linked with the condition. People with sleep apnoea tend to feel sluggish and low-spirited all the time. In the medium term, sleep apnoea can cause a lowering of the metabolic rate, leading to obesity – so obesity can be a result, as well as a cause, of the condition.

In the long term, episodes of sleep apnoea lead to the brain becoming starved of oxygen, which, in its turn, can lead to fluctuations in heart rate as adrenalin pours into the bloodstream to wake the sleeper. This can speed up the heartbeat, making it more irregular, which can be dangerous for anyone with an underlying heart condition. People with sleep apnoea also tend to have higher blood pressure. Research studies in the USA, Canada and Israel have all shown that high blood pressure is associated with breathing pauses during sleep – exactly what happens in sleep apnoea.

An American doctor, speaking at the British Sleep Society conference in Edinburgh in 1997, suggested that the higher an individual's blood pressure, the more episodes of apnoea they will have, and that people who have more than five respiratory disturbances per hour are likely to develop high blood pressure. High blood pressure is, of course, a risk factor for later stroke illness as well as vascular disease, angina and heart attacks. Quite a high proportion of heart attacks occur at night, during sleep, and may be precipitated, if not actually caused, by sleep apnoea. One ENT surgeon compares breathing when you have a blocked airway to trying to push a car up a slope. It demands great effort and puts a strain on the heart, which is not good news for anyone with heart problems.

Diagnosing sleep apnoea

How would you know if you had sleep apnoea? Severe and persistent daytime sleepiness – not just tiredness – is the most obvious symptom, since many sufferers are not really aware of the obstruction–choking–breathing cycles they may go through during the night. Doctors say that it is often a partner who is the first to realize that the sufferer has something more than just a severe snoring problem. If you already know that you snore, and you are feeling continually exhausted, prone to dropping off over the newspaper or in front of the TV, you might suspect sleep apnoea. If you're the sort of person who falls asleep any time, anywhere – at work, over dinner, even, most frighteningly of all, at the wheel of your car – don't delay, go to your GP straight away and check whether sleep apnoea is at the root of the problem.

The sleep study

In order for a diagnosis of sleep apnoea to be confirmed you will probably have to take part in a 'sleep study', either in a specialized sleep study unit or under the care of a hospital lung specialist. A sleep study normally involves an overnight stay in hospital and a variety of painless tests so that the medical staff can tell how badly your breathing is obstructed and your sleep disturbed. You will probably have to wear special belts around your chest and stomach in order to monitor your breathing, and a clip attached to your finger to measure the amount of oxygen in your blood. Sometimes the medical team will use video to check your body movements and the quality of your sleep. Tests will include:

- simple visual observation, to detect the signs of sleep apnoea, like laboured breathing with long pauses followed by arousal from sleep;
- pulse oximetry, which measures the amount of oxygen in the blood, and the pulse rate. People with sleep apnoea are found to have multiple 'dips' in oxygen level and peaks in pulse rate;
- polysomnography, which measures eye movements and chin tone in order to see which sleep stage the sleeper has reached. The flow of air through the nose and mouth, the movement of the chest wall, and the oxygen levels in the blood, are also measured. In a normal sleeper, the breathing is regular and rhythmic, the heart rate is stable, and the oxygen saturation in the blood is 95 per cent. During an episode of sleep apnoea, the level of oxygen in the blood quickly begins to decline to a low level, there are gaps in the airflow at least once a minute, and within 30 seconds the heart rate begins to rise and breathing starts again;
- an ECG (electrocardiograph) to measure any seriously abnormal heart rhythms.

Another way of assessing sleep quality that can be done in your own home has been pioneered by the British Lung Foundation, using a method called Pulse Transit Time, or PTT. This is an indirect way of measuring blood pressure and provides information about airway narrowing and sleep disturbance, using a small portable device that can be used in the sufferer's own home, rather than in a sleep laboratory.

Treatment

At the moment it is not known why some snorers go on to develop sleep apnoea. It may be that patients who develop this condition have larger tongues or short lower jaws in addition to the other risk factors like being overweight. Simple lifestyle changes such as those recommended in Chapter 3 may help to reduce the symptoms. Certainly, the overweight and heavy drinkers seem to be more at risk. The shape of the jaw has an influence too. 'Retrograde jaw structure' – otherwise known as the 'chinless wonder' look – can predispose an individual towards sleep apnoea. Dental devices like the Snore Guard, which holds the jaw forward, preventing the chin and any surrounding tissue from restricting the airway, can also be effective in preventing it. The most common type of anti-snoring surgery, UPPP, or uvulo-palato-pharyngoplasty (see Chapter 5), is now only used in the tiny minority of sleep apnoea sufferers who can't or won't use a CPAP machine. However, some surgeons are now claiming that the use of a fibre-optic device called a nasendoscope to inspect the nasal cavity can make surgery more effective.

The most effective treatment in current use is the CPAP machine (see Chapter 4). The slightly pressurized air pumped into the nose and throat by these machines does keep the airway open. A CPAP machine begins to work as soon as you put it on and it helps most patients, as many as 99 per cent, who are able to enjoy a night of restful sleep and function effectively in the daytime. The disadvantages of the machine are that it is rather expensive and cumbersome. Sleeping with a mask over most of your face and a pump beside the bed may not be an ideal solution, but many patients and partners feel that it is a price worth paying for uninterrupted slumbers. Sleep apnoea is not only miserable for the sufferer, who is continually exhausted and lacking in energy, but also for the partner, who finds it impossible to sleep. It's also life-threatening, so getting used to a CPAP machine may literally be the only option.

Successful treatment: Philip and Alan

Philip is 55 and has been treated for sleep apnoea for five years:

My wife recognized that I had a problem before I did. I snored really noisily and it affected the whole family. I managed to give up smoking a few years ago, which I thought might help, but it didn't. I suppose, if I'm honest, I admit that I could do with losing some weight. I did try to diet and lost a stone at one point but it didn't make any difference to my snoring problem. The children used to complain about it as well as my wife. I thought I was sleeping all right, but before I was diagnosed with sleep apnoea I felt tired during the day and would fall asleep as soon as I came in from work in the evening.

It was after I dozed off at the traffic lights when I was driving home from work one day that I decided that I really ought to see someone about it, although I honestly didn't think that anything could be done.

My GP referred me to the chest clinic at the local hospital which surprised me for a start, because I never thought I had a chest problem. They had all sorts of equipment that they tested me with. They asked me how often I woke up during the night and tested the oxygen levels in my blood, because apparently having reduced oxygen levels leads to health complications in the long term.

Eventually they told me I had sleep apnoea, which I had never heard of before. I now have a CPAP machine and I honestly wouldn't be without it. I felt awkward using it at first, because I have to wear a mask at night and the machine pumps air into my nose so it takes a bit of time to get used to. It was worth it, though, because my wife and I both got a good night's sleep for the first time for years.

My machine goes everywhere with me, including Australia and the USA on holiday. I don't want to risk the embarrassment I suffered before. We once went on a holiday to Turkey on one of those boats, a *gulet*, where you sleep in tiny cabins, and I kept the whole boat awake with my snoring. That's all in the past now. I don't feel tired in the daytime any more and my general health has improved.

Alan, whose marriage broke up because of his snoring problem, has been using a CPAP machine for nine months and calls it a life-saver:

> It is cumbersome, but it enables me to have about six hours of quality sleep a night and that has made a huge difference. It takes some time to get used to the machine. The nasal mask is held on with straps and if you wear them too tight it hurts, but if they aren't tight enough the mask doesn't fit snugly over your face. Then having cold air blowing over your face at night can keep you awake in itself, and there's the question of maintaining the machine and making sure it's working properly. In spite of the disadvantages, though, it does seem to help me sleep more quietly. While I was having the sleep study done, there was another young man in the unit whose snores were absolutely deafening, so I can appreciate what my ex-wife went through.

If your partner notices you apparently gasping for breath, choking and stopping breathing as you snore, and you are exhausted, drowsy, lethargic, forgetful, moody and irritable during the daytime, your problem could be sleep apnoea, rather than simple snoring. Don't delay if this is the case: enlist the help of your GP who will refer you for a sleep study. Of course, there's nothing to stop you making those necessary lifestyle changes (see Chapter 3) – losing some weight, stopping smoking and reducing your alcohol consumption – while you wait.

8

Don't Forget the Snoree!

Snoring is one of the few health problems that arguably causes more difficulties for the sufferer's partner, family and friends than it does for the sufferer himself. Some snorers genuinely don't believe they have a serious problem until they hear themselves on tape. Snoring can lead to a complete breakdown in relationships. No one is at their most loving and tolerant when they are not getting enough sleep. If a partner feels that the snorer is not taking the issue seriously, or is unwilling to go for help, it can drive a wedge between even the most loving couples.

'I just lie there at night, desperate to go off to sleep before Mike does because I know if he starts snoring I haven't a hope,' says one wife:

> Even on the rare occasions when he is sleeping quietly, I'm on edge because I don't know when he is going to start up again. I spend part of four or five nights every week in the spare room, or on the living-room sofa where I am out of earshot. I feel uncomfortable, resentful, and above all, exhausted. As for our love life, forget it. Most of the time I am just too tired to bother.

Snoring can and does lead to divorce – not often by itself, but as a symbol of deeper problems in the relationship. It's not just that you are both exhausted. If he doesn't care enough to seek treatment, if he's turned into a slob who slumps in front on the TV every evening, it's easy to think he doesn't really care at all. And snoring can be a problem in new relationships too. What happens if you have recently met and want to spend a night together? Your partner can book a romantic hotel with a four-poster bed, a candle-lit dinner, champagne . . . but the atmosphere is going to be less than romantic if he snores.

A recent survey of 1,000 British couples found that more than half had argued about snoring and one couple in ten had even considered splitting up! Some of the survey's other findings were that:

- eight out of ten partners frequently or always find it difficult to get to sleep because of their partner's snoring;

- 66 per cent always or frequently lie awake at night;
- 73 per cent say they always or frequently feel tired the next morning;
- 54 per cent say they always or frequently feel stressed and emotional;
- 30 per cent feel their work suffers as a result of their partner's snoring;
- 39 per cent of snorers and 33 per cent of partners felt that snoring has adversely affected their relationship;
- 25 per cent of snorers and 22 per cent of partners believe that snoring has adversely affected their sex life.

What can snorees do?

Most of these statistics will not be news to the partners and families of snorers. What, apart from earplugs or divorce, can partners – or 'snorees', as they are sometimes known – do to help? After all, it may not be the snorer's fault that he has a problem and he is not doing it to annoy you. According to the BSSAA, they are approached for help as frequently by the partners of snorers as by the snorers themselves.

If you are a snoree, there are two ways to deal with it. One, by getting your partner to admit he needs help, and two, to get some help yourself. Recognize that snoring is not a joke, or something you have to tolerate, but that sleep deprivation is actually harmful and that you need sleep as much as your partner does. Laboratory rats die after being deprived of sleep for 14 days. Lack of proper sleep, particularly over a period of time, can cause genuine health problems. You will find yourself becoming irritable and easily upset. Sleeplessness also affects your concentration and attention span. Complex tasks like operating machinery or driving are more difficult for the sleep-deprived. You may also feel anxious and even unreal, a phenomenon known as depersonalization. You could suffer from muscle tension and headaches as well as the more obvious symptoms of tiredness like lack of energy. Palpitations, panic attacks, increased susceptibility to colds and minor infections, even high blood pressure and stomach ulcers have all been suggested as possible effects of lack of sleep. It's not selfish or self-indulgent to understand that *your partner's* snoring can be *your* problem, too.

Tell the experts

GPs, ENT specialists and sleep clinics all welcome input from the snoree when they are deciding on a diagnosis. After all, you are the one who actually hears the snoring, night after night, and the more detail you can give the doctors about it, the easier it becomes for useful treatment to be prescribed. A specialist will want to know:

- if the snoring is continuous, or comes and goes;
- if the snoring only happens when the snorer is lying on his back, and whether his mouth is open or closed;
- what sorts of sounds he makes;
- if he seems to gasp for breath, or even stop breathing, which would indicate that he suffers from sleep apnoea rather than simple snoring.

Often, this is information only a partner can give.

Try earplugs

Earplugs, which you can buy from any good chemist, are one obvious solution for the desperate snoree, although no earplugs are going to mask the sound of a truly heroic snorer sleeping a foot away from you! One ENT surgeon I spoke to recommended gun shops as a good source of high-quality earplugs. Apparently there are companies who produce tailor-made earplugs, from a mould rather like the one used to make a hearing aid, which will be comfortable and won't fall out during the night.

The BSSAA sell a range of earplugs, including some which are disposable and others which come with their own cleaning solution, but emphasize that even the best earplugs are not going to drown out the sounds of snoring completely.

'Top-of-the-range earplugs might reduce snoring by around 30 decibels, but as most severe snorers produce 50-plus decibels and many a lot more than that, earplugs are not a complete answer,' says the Association's Marianne Davey. 'Our advice to partners is to work with the snorer to find a solution to the problem. Partners can often tell us what the snorer can't.'

Among the earplugs available from the BSSAA are Sleep Soft earplugs, which have two filters, allowing the user to select the most suitable level of noise reduction, and come with their own carrying case. Eski earplugs, apparently one of the BSSAA's best-sellers, are made of foam. Mack's Pillow Soft silicone earplugs from the USA are said to mould easily to the ear and don't crackle like some earplugs. Mack's also make Ear Seals (basically, earplugs with a removable cord) and a special smaller-size set of earplugs for children. All these earplugs claim to reduce snoring noise by between 22 and 28 decibels.

Use stress reduction techniques

Stress reduction techniques can help you deal with the edgy, irritable feeling. See Chapter 6 for information about complementary therapies for this. Both Bach Flower Remedies and hypnotherapy are recommended to help snorees. Traditional Chinese medicine believes that sleep is a natural tonic and ancient Chinese texts recommend sleeping 'like a bow' with your body curled up on your right side, so that your heart is higher up. Washing your feet in a basin of warm water before bed is also supposed to help you sleep. According to Feng Shui principles your bedhead should face east in spring and summer and west in autumn and winter to ensure sound sleep!

Sleeplessness, however it's caused, is one of those issues that soon becomes a vicious circle. The more you worry about not being able to sleep, the more wakeful you are. Once you convince yourself that the moment you get into bed your partner will start to snore, you will inevitably tense up and sleep will elude you. Psychologist Ken Gibbons says that it's important to address the problem with your partner before it becomes a serious issue, even if this means tackling it in the early stages of a relationship:

> So many people wait until they are driven crazy by a partner's personal habits, including snoring, and then shout at them. Quite often the reaction from the partner is 'Why didn't you say something before? Why didn't you tell me?' It's never easy to find a tactful way to bring the subject up, though you could try mentioning a fictional friend's snoring problem. The important thing is to communicate and try to deal with it together, before it destroys the relationship.

Aim for a good night's sleep

Sometimes going to bed well before your partner can help – you will be fast asleep before his thunderous snores can wake you. That old traditional standby, a milky drink, can be soothing. Milk contains tryptophan, which is converted during digestion into a substance that helps the brain to produce sleep hormones. Daytime exercise will mean you are pleasantly physically tired at bedtime, but don't exercise too late in the evening. Exercise can produce adrenalin, which keeps you awake, as do stimulants like tea and coffee. Instead, wind down slowly with some undemanding TV or a good book, followed by a warm bath with the addition of some calming aromatherapy oils like camomile, lavender or sandalwood.

Don't rely on an alcoholic nightcap or sleeping pills to ensure you get a good night's sleep. Alcohol is a depressant and although you might drop off after a few drinks, you are quite likely to wake in the small hours to hear your partner snoring. Sleeping pills are not really appropriate for a long-term difficulty like having a snoring partner. They are usually only prescribed to enable you to re-establish a good sleeping habit and your GP will normally suggest a short course of the lowest possible effective dose. Apart from the risks of dependency, there is some evidence that drug-induced sleep is not the same as normal sleep. Studies of sleep patterns show that sleepers experience less dream sleep and less really deep sleep after taking medication. If you take sleeping pills for a long time, withdrawal can lead to much longer periods of dream sleep, sometimes causing nightmares. It's better to encourage natural sleep by using any relaxation method that works for you, from meditation to deep-breathing exercises. Visualization can help too – imagine yourself walking down the steps into a beautiful, tranquil garden or along a sunlit beach. Gentle, New Age-style music and relaxation tapes and CDs are widely available and can work for some people.

Face relationship problems

Marriage guidance counsellors are used to the subject of snoring coming up as an issue between couples with relationship problems. 'It is something that people argue about, like leaving the loo seat up,' says Relate spokesperson Julia Cole:

It may be linked to other issues like excessive drinking or being overweight and the non-snoring partner may feel that the snorer is doing it deliberately. What I would do is look underneath and ask if the partner was really worried about the snorer's drinking or bad eating habits. The trouble is that snoring is somehow associated with piggery, self-indulgence and general slobbish habits. It's sometimes difficult for couples to discuss it without the snorer feeling he is being got at. It's important for the partner not to nag and criticize. Snoring can be caused by the shape of the snorer's palate, or the position he sleeps in, not by being a slob! Putting your partner's back up will only make him feel hurt and angry. Supporting him by saying that you will come to the doctor with him because you're worried can be much more helpful.

Make him feel you are on his side in tackling the snoring, rather than accusing him or snapping at him to 'do something about it' before stamping off to the spare room!

It is important to deal with snoring in the same way that you would any other relationship difficulty – by talking about it and agreeing to seek help if you can, rather than by accusation and criticism. If the snorer does have a problem with obesity, drinking or smoking, you could agree to give up smoking or join a gym or start a healthy eating plan *together*.

What about the snorer who won't admit there's a problem or agree to seek help?

'You might have to resort to taping the snores or enlisting the support of the family or the rest of the household,' says Julia. 'Again, try to be tactful. The last thing you should do is shame the snorer among his friends at work or in the pub, which will only make him embarrassed and defensive. Keep it within the family.'

She adds that fear may be involved too. 'Men are notoriously unwilling to go to the doctor. Joining a self-help organization like the BSSAA and getting information from them could be a starting point.'

Keep romance alive!

If you and your partner decide that while he is still snoring separate bedrooms are the only solution, it is possible to keep your relationship alive and healthy. After all, the aristocracy, with their large houses, have slept in separate rooms for centuries and still managed to have sex lives and large families. In fact, at one time it was regarded as rather vulgar for married couples to share a bedroom. It was what poor people who couldn't afford anything else had to do.

'Don't feel that it is a failure of love if you can't put up with someone's snoring,' says Julia:

If you move to the spare room, you are saying that you need a good night's rest, not that you want to punish your partner for something that, after all, is not his fault. Make sure he knows that.

Some couples prefer to sleep in separate rooms for all sorts of reasons. However, if you are used to being together, separate rooms can make you feel isolated, alienated, and as if the snorer is being punished. Unless you make a real effort to keep the intimacy alive, it can drive a wedge between you.

If you do sleep separately, it's important to show each other as much physical affection as possible when you are together. Kisses, hugs and holding hands really matter. If you don't actually sleep together, you might need to be more upfront about when you feel like a cuddle or sex, rather than just waiting for it to happen 'naturally'. You will need to be open and talk about it and perhaps plan to visit one another on Friday night.

You could even make a romance, a 'date' of it. Make it fun. Set the scene with low lights, music, perhaps candles, so that it feels exciting and different rather than an admission of failure. You could even explore each other's fantasies by pretending you are in a hotel room or whatever turns you on.

You *can* maintain a loving relationship sleeping in separate rooms, but you need to put some thought into it if it's to be a permanent arrangement. The problems arise if one partner feels banished or is stuck on an uncomfortable camp bed in a tiny spare room. You need to be creative and make sure the room you sleep in is just as homely and comfortable as the main bedroom. I've heard of couples where one partner sleeps in the children's room, but this isn't a good idea. It's telling children too much about their parents' relationship. It can make the snoring partner feel ganged up on, and confuses the children.

Coping with snoring

Sue and Greg

Sue and Greg have been married for 30 years, though it is only in the last 10 that Greg's snoring has caused them real problems. They have decided that separate bedrooms are the only solution.

Sue says that, to begin with, she would just nudge Greg when he started snoring and he would turn over and stop:

But when it got to the point when every breath he took was a snore, I was getting no sleep at all. I have had two non-sleeping babies so I knew what it was like to suffer from sleep deprivation, with the inevitable tiredness and irritability. I was willing to try anything. Sometimes he doesn't seem to be breathing, which troubles me. I lie there thinking that perhaps I should wake him up, but then he starts to snore again. Either way, sleep is out of the question.

I remember the first really bad night, because we were on a ski-ing holiday. We'd had an exhausting day on the slopes. Greg slept like the dead, but he snored so loudly that I ended up sleeping in the bath – because, of course, in a hotel room you have no alternative.

I experimented with various kinds of earplugs. Most were not very helpful and left me with a sort of roaring sound in my ears. I did find some in Australia which are made of some kind of soft, malleable silicone; I'm not sure if you can get them in Britain. If Greg and I do share a bed I wear them and take half a sleeping tablet as well, but I wouldn't want to do that on a permanent basis. Wearing earplugs for too long gives me ear infections and I don't want to become dependent on tablets.

Greg must have tried just about every preparation and device on the market and we have found them all more or less useless. He is not a good sleeper anyway, perhaps because his job means that he travels extensively and crosses a lot of time zones. He seems exhausted a lot of the time. If we go out in the evening it's not unknown for him to fall asleep in the theatre or at the ballet and I dread him starting to snore. I did buy him a device like a wrist-watch that I saw in Harrods' technology department, which was supposed to vibrate when he snored and wake him up. When he tried it I did get a good night's sleep but it woke him up so often he hardly got any sleep at all!

We haven't had much help from the medical profession. Greg was referred to an ENT specialist who more or less told him to come back when he had lost some weight and then he could try one of those CPAP machines. He is quite heavily built and we both understand that snoring is linked to weight, but he has honestly been trying to lose it ever since we married. We eat a very healthy, Mediterranean-type diet, with plenty of fruit and veg, and he probably eats less than I do. I don't see how he could eat less without starving! I felt that the doctors could have been more sympathetic. No one sets out to be fat.

We both know that surgery might help but are reluctant to go that far – so, at present, separate rooms are the only way we can both sleep. When I slept in the same room I used to feel murderous and shout at him, then he would shout back, so we are better sleeping on our own. I feel guilty that it's necessary, and we both miss the closeness and intimacy of sleeping together, but we don't feel there is any alternative. We have a good relationship and a long marriage, in spite of the snoring.

Melanie

Melanie feels that her eight-year relationship with her boyfriend has been affected by his snoring problem, which neither of them have managed to come to terms with. They don't share a home, and 'staying over' is a different prospect when they can't spend a whole night together:

There is definitely less physical closeness, less intimacy, between us because of it. I don't mind sleeping alone and it's certainly worth creeping into his spare room when he starts snoring, but I know he misses me. I have noticed that it's harder for us to make up a quarrel or even a difference of opinion, because we don't have that relaxed, cuddly feeling couples have when they wake up in the same bed. If we're not careful, unless we make a point of holding hands in the street and so on, the only physical contact we have is when we are actually making love, and I don't think that's satisfactory for either of us.

When I do stay in his spare room I have trained myself to wake up early in the morning and sneak back into his bed before he wakes up so that at least we don't miss out on a cuddle.

Christine

Holidays can be a major problem for snorees, with no living-room sofa or comfortable spare room to escape to. The confined space of a tent or caravan can mean misery for the whole family, not to mention the neighbours. Apartment-sharing is not an option. Like Sue, whose story is told above, and who ended up sleeping in the bath, Christine had problems on holiday with her snoring husband. 'In the end I became so frustrated that I wrapped myself in a blanket and went to sleep in the hotel corridor,' she admits. 'It was very embarrassing being woken by the cleaner at 6 a.m., but our room only had a shower, not a bath, so what choice did I have?'

Christine's husband broke his nose some years ago and his snoring is thought to be nose-based. They are currently investigating the possibility of surgery.

Tackle the problem together

There can be little doubt about it, snoring does adversely affect relationships. It may seem a trivial problem to those on the outside but however much you care for someone, living in a permanent state of sleep deprivation puts a strain on even the most loving partnership. The only way to cope is to tackle it – as you would any relationship difficulty – together. Admit you have a problem, if you're the snorer. Accept that he isn't doing it to annoy you, if you're the snoree. Be supportive in the search for a cure and take good care of your own health. If that means you have to sleep separately for a while, make sure the snorer knows that it's not because you don't love him and care about him. It's a lot easier to treat someone with love and understanding if you're not half-dead from exhaustion . . .

9
Further Help

Having got this far, I hope you are convinced that snoring matters. It's not a joke, either for the snorer or for his (or her) long-suffering partner, family, flatmates – or even those unlucky enough to have the next room in the thinly walled holiday hotel. Snoring can wreck relationships and leave families exhausted and stressed-out. Sleep apnoea, bluntly, can kill. In the USA, daytime sleepiness has been estimated to cost the country a massive $16 billion, with over 200,000 road accidents the result of lack of sleep. The good news is that you don't have to suffer any of this. Even the most seemingly intractable snoring problem can be treated, usually by a combination of self-help and medical intervention.

Helping yourself

Recognize the problem
The first thing any snorer has to do is recognize the problem. If you can't hear yourself, others can, and it's in no one's interest to deny that you snore. Finding out what is making you snore may be a simple matter or it may involve a great deal of trial and error, but the answer is there somewhere. All you have to do is find it.

You may be lucky and find that one of the over-the-counter, easily available snoring remedies works for you, perhaps because you have been suffering from nasal congestion or a flabby soft palate that is tightened up by one of the many sprays on the market. More likely, though, there will be no overnight cure. Lifestyle changes will undoubtedly help – all snoring experts agree that if you lose weight, stop smoking and cut down on your drinking, your snoring is likely to improve whether you have any other treatment or not. Dropping one collar size – say, from a size 17 to a size 16 – is likely to have a noticeable effect on your snoring. Both palatal surgery and dental devices are more effective on slim people than they are on fat ones. Your snoring could be caused by a combination of factors and you'll need to tackle all of them to see results.

Start with the obvious
Eliminate the obvious possibilities first. If you are overweight, start a

new healthy eating and fitness regime. Yes, today – what are you waiting for? If you are a heavy drinker, at least cut down, or restrict your drinking to lunchtimes and early evenings, leaving a gap of at least four hours between drinking any alcohol and going to bed. If you are a smoker, give up. If you have a permanently stuffed-up nose and catarrh, investigate the possibility of an allergy, perhaps caused by something common like house-dust mites or pet hair, or by something you are eating.

Try the simple remedies suggested in Chapter 3, like sleeping with a pillow in the small of your back or raising the head of the bed. You might also like to try one of the many over-the-counter throat sprays on the market to tone up those flabby throat muscles.

See your GP

Enlist the help of your GP and don't be afraid you are wasting her time. She will probably suggest the self-help measures you have already tried, but if they haven't worked she should be willing to refer you to an ENT specialist or sleep studies unit. There are several hundred of these around the country and waiting times vary. You might also mention the problem to your dentist to see if there is anything unusual about the shape of your jaw that might be causing the problems. You'll need to give your GP, dentist and specialist all the information you can – enlisting the help of your partner if you have one – for them to be able to arrive at an accurate diagnosis. Your problem may turn out to be simple snoring, or if you are excessively sleepy during the daytime and your partner reports episodes of breathlessness and choking during the night, you might learn that you have sleep apnoea.

Once you have been diagnosed, your doctors will recommend the most appropriate treatment, which could be anything from a specially designed mandibular advancement device you wear in your mouth, to laser or conventional surgery, to a CPAP machine that keeps your airway open by blowing air into your nose and throat as you sleep. Whether you have started to snore relatively recently or have been a snorer for years, you can still be treated, so don't give up.

Helping agencies

Details of all the agencies and helplines listed in this section can be found in Useful Addresses, p. 83.

The BSSAA

Remember that you are not alone. You will certainly find it helpful to join the 40,000 members of the British Snoring and Sleep Apnoea Association (BSSAA). Their helpline number is 0800 085 1097, and they also have a comprehensive website. The BSSAA have years of experience in advising snorers and their partners and are always up to date on the latest research. They have a regular newsletter, test all the advertised 'snoring cures' that appear on the market, and they also offer tips and hints from members on everything from travelling with your CPAP machine to how to calculate your BMI or body-mass index (the figure that tells you if you are overweight, see p. 20). One of their most useful leaflets details their '90-Day Snore-no-More Plan', which sets out in the form of a diagram the steps you should take to analyse your problem and then solve it.

Sleep apnoea

If you have been diagnosed with sleep apnoea you might also benefit from contacting the Sleep Apnoea Trust, tel. 01494 527772. They don't offer medical help, simply practical advice from other sufferers. They help fund research, organize conferences and produce a Medical Alert card that warns doctors and paramedics that you have sleep apnoea, in case of an emergency.

The British Lung Foundation is also involved in research and providing information about sleep apnoea, including a free leaflet. They also have a network of 120 Breathe Easy clubs around the country aimed at supporting people with breathing problems. For details of your nearest, contact the BLF on 020 7831 5831.

Allergies

If you suspect that an allergy may be at the root of your snoring problem, contact Allergy UK, tel. 020 8303 8583, who can give you details about where to buy things like anti-allergy bed-linen and vacuum cleaners with special filters to deal with pet hair, house-dust mites and other common allergens. Companies specializing in this sort of equipment include Medivac on 0845 130 6969 and Medibed on 01282 839700. Allergy UK can also give information about testing for food allergies.

Healthy eating and losing weight

For more information about healthy eating, including details of the special Lighten Up workshops for men who are interested in losing weight safely and permanently, call 0845 603 3456. If you haven't exercised for years, don't embark on a new fitness regime without having a word with your GP, and make sure you take things slowly at first.

Smoking and alcohol

There's no easy way to give up smoking and you will need willpower, but for help in saying goodbye to the deadly weed call Quitline on 0800 002 200. If you suspect that heavy drinking – more than the recommended level of 3–4 units a day for men or 2–3 units a day for women – could be part of the problem, help is available from Alcoholics Anonymous, helpline 0845 7697 555, or the Alcohol Concern helpline on 0800 917 8282. Both organizations welcome enquiries from anyone concerned about their drinking. If it's your partner's alcohol intake that is causing concern, call Al-Anon on 020 7403 0888. Please also bear in mind that you don't have to drink up to these maximum recommended levels to have a snoring problem. Even small amounts of alcohol could be enough to relax the muscles in your throat.

Complementary therapies

If you would like to find out more about what complementary therapies have to offer, make sure that the practitioners you consult are members of the relevant professional organization and are properly qualified. The organizations listed in Useful Addresses (p. 84) will be able to advise you and put you in touch with a local therapist.

What about the future?

Ear, nose and throat specialists and snoring experts are, inevitably, concerned about the increase in obesity in Britain. Estimates vary, but it has been said that by 2010 as many as half of the population could be obese, or 30 per cent above the recommended weight for their height. More obese people, sadly, means more snorers, and more pressure on the facilities available to treat them.

Michael Timms, consultant ENT surgeon at the Abbey Gisburne Park Hospital in Lancashire, says that what is needed is a method of widening the airway side to side, as a CPAP machine does, as well as front to back.

'When we do a scan and we see the throat moving we can see the airway is blocked in both dimensions,' he explains. 'We need to find a way of stretching the whole airway!'

Grant Bates from the Radcliffe Infirmary in Oxford points out that ENT specialists are trying new techniques all the time:

> Harmonic scalpels are a useful advance because they cut down the pain involved in surgery. One British surgeon at Cambridge was copying a technique that had been used in the USA, where they tend to do more surgery for snoring problems than we do here. With this particular technique, a sort of paste was injected into the palate to stiffen it. The initial results were quite good but he did a follow-up study on the patients and found that after two years the success rate had fallen from 80 per cent to 40 per cent. There are always innovations in treatments but the safest way to reduce snoring is simply to lose weight.

CPAP machines, the treatment of choice for sleep apnoea and some severe snorers, are becoming increasingly sophisticated as well as smaller and more user-friendly. In the early 1980s the average machine was the size of a small fridge, while the most recent models are no bigger than a book. Some can be linked via a modem to the computer in a sleep laboratory, enabling doctors to monitor exactly what is happening to a patient's airways during sleep and providing a computer print-out if required. Traditional CPAP units are set to the appropriate pressure for the individual patient by the hospital or sleep laboratory after a sleep study. Auto-CPAP machines have their own built-in memory and are able to alter the pressure according to the patient's needs during periods of sleep. Masks are also being improved all the time and there are now gel masks that mould to the face, special 'nose pillows' and 'breathe headgear', all intended to make use of the machine more comfortable and as unobtrusive as possible.

Dr John Rees of Guy's Hospital says that future developments in snoring treatments are likely to include further development of CPAP machines, simpler devices for mandibular advancement, and possibly electrical stimulation devices to increase the action of specific throat muscles.

Marianne Davey of the BSSAA doesn't think that there will be a breakthrough in the way snoring is treated in the foreseeable future, but that the current products on the market will continue to be refined and improved:

Treatments are being updated all the time. As the BSSAA becomes more high-profile we get more calls from doctors and hospitals as well as snorers and their partners. We attend lots of training days and seminars aimed at spreading the word throughout the medical profession. As far as snorers are concerned we are totally unbiased towards any particular form of treatment; we simply set out the facts as we know them and then leave people to make up their own minds what to try.

Snoring is very much an individual problem, with individual solutions. What works for one person won't necessarily work for the next. Finding a cure takes time. The remedy is out there, somewhere, if you have the patience to seek it out and the determination to find it, making whatever lifestyle changes are necessary to ensure silent, snore-free nights. Sweet dreams!

Top ten tips for silent nights . . . for snorers

1 Admit that you snore.
2 If you're overweight, lose those excess kilos.
3 If you smoke, quit.
4 If you're a drinker, cut down, and don't drink within four hours of bedtime.
5 Try to work out why you snore, following the tests on p. 14.
6 Join the BSSAA.
7 Enlist the help of your partner and family, who may be able to tell you whether or not you have the symptoms of sleep apnoea.
8 Go to your GP, armed with the information you already have.
9 If simple lifestyle changes and over-the-counter medicines have not helped, ask if you can be referred for a sleep study.
10 The results of the sleep study should show whether you are a heavy snorer who would benefit from surgery or a mandibular advancement device, or whether you suffer from sleep apnoea, for which a CPAP machine is the treatment of choice.

Top ten tips for silent nights . . . for partners

1 Recognize that you have a problem. However much you love your snoring partner, you still need to sleep.
2 Try to separate the way you feel about the person from the way you feel about the snoring. They are not doing it to annoy you.

3 Express concern rather than anger.
4 Don't tease them about it, particularly not in public.
5 If they refuse to seek help, see if you can find out why. They may, for instance, be terrified of surgery, and you can reassure them that there are other treatment options.
6 When they do see the GP or specialist, go with them. Your input will be invaluable in diagnosing the exact problem.
7 Take especial care of your own health. Practise relaxation techniques and catch up on your sleep whenever you can.
8 Earplugs and early nights – so that you get to sleep before your partner does – are worth a try.
9 Encourage your partner to make lifestyle changes by joining in.
10 If you decide separate rooms are the answer, even temporarily, make sure it's clearly understood that you are avoiding the snoring, not rejecting your partner!

Useful Addresses

All types of snoring

British Snoring and Sleep Apnoea Association (BSSAA)
2nd Floor Suite
52 Albert Road North
Reigate
Surrey RH2 9EL
Helpline: 0800 085 1097
Website: <www.britishsnoring.co.uk>

Sleep apnoea

British Lung Foundation
78 Hatton Garden
London EC1N 8JR
Tel: 020 7831 5831
Website: <www.lunguk.org>

Sleep Apnoea Trust
7 Bailey Close
High Wycombe HP13 6QA
Tel: 01494 527772
Website: <www.sleep-apnoea-trust.org>

Allergies

Allergy UK
Deepdene House
30 Bellegrove Road
Welling
Kent DA16 3PY
Tel: 020 8303 8583
Website: <www.allergyuk.org>

Medibed
Tel: 01282 839700

Medivac
Tel: 0845 130 6969
Website: <www.medivac.co.uk>

Healthy living

Al-Anon
61 Great Dover Street
London SE1 4YF
Tel: 020 7403 0888
Website: <www.hexnet.co.uk/alanon/>

Alcohol Concern
Waterbridge House
32–36 Loman Street
London SE1 0EE
Helpline: 0800 917 8282
Website: <www.alcoholconcern.org.uk>

Alcoholics Anonymous
PO Box 1
Stonebow House
Stonebow
York YO1 7NJ
Helpline: 0845 7697 555
Website: <www.alcoholics-anonymous.org.uk>

Boots 'Lifestyle Programmes'
Tel: 0845 120 3000

Lighten Up Workshops
46 Staines Road
Twickenham TW2 5AH
Tel: 0845 603 3456
Website: <www.lightenup.co.uk>

Quitline
Helpline: 0800 002 200
Website: <www.quit.org.uk>
For help in giving up smoking

Complementary therapies

AcuMedic Centre
101–105 Camden High Street
London NW1 7JN
Tel: 020 7388 6704
Website: <www.acumedic.com>
Specialists in traditional Chinese medicine

Acupuncture Council
63 Jeddo Road
London W12 9QH
Tel: 020 8735 0400
Website: <www.acupuncture.org.uk>

Ayurvedic Medical Association UK
1079 Garratt Lane
London SW17 0LN
Tel: 020 8682 3876

Bach Flower Remedies
The Bach Centre
Mount Vernon
Sotwell
Oxfordshire OX10 0PZ
Tel: 01491 834678
Website: <www.bachcentre.com>

British Homoeopathic Association
15 Clerkenwell Close
London EC1R 0AA
Tel: 020 7566 7800
Helpline: 09065 343404
Website: <www.trusthomeopathy.org>

British Society for Clinical Hypnosis
c/o Tom Connelly
125 Queensgate
Bridlington YO16 7JQ
Tel: 020 7499 2813 or 01262 403103
Website: <www.bsch.org.uk>

British Wheel of Yoga
25 Jermyn Street
Sleaford
Lincolnshire NG34 7RU
Tel: 01529 306851
Website: <www.bwy.org.uk>

Chi Health Centres
Helpline: 020 7233 5566 (Monday to Saturday)
Website: <www.chihealthcentres.com>
Health centres that combine traditional and complementary medicines
with psychology, and offer advice with no obligation or commitment
via their helpline

The Hale Clinic
7 Park Crescent
London W1N 3HE
Tel: 020 7631 0156
Website: <www.haleclinic.com>

Homoeopathic Helpline
Tel: 09065 343404

Integrated Medical Centre
43 New Cavendish Street
London W1G 9TH
Tel: 020 7224 5111
Website: <www.integratedmedical.co.uk>

National Institute of Medical Herbalists
56 Longbrook Street
Exeter
Devon EX4 6AH
Tel: 01392 426022
Website: <www.nimh.org.uk>

Sara Rossi
99 Sinclair Road
London W14 0NP
Tel: 020 7602 3967
Email: rossi_sara@hotmail.com
Registered homoeopath and British Wheel of Yoga teacher

Society of Teachers of the Alexander Technique
129 Camden Mews
London NW1 9AH
Tel: 020 7382 5159
Website: <www.stat.org.uk>

Index

INDEX